Communicating with Children and their Families

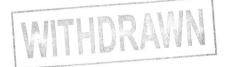

Communicating with Children and their Families

Responding to need and protection

Liz Davies and Evelyn Kerrigan Lebloch

 Open University Press

Open University Press
McGraw-Hill Education
McGraw-Hill House
Shoppenhangers Road
Maidenhead
Berkshire
England
SL6 2QL

email: enquiries@openup.co.uk
world wide web: www.openup.co.uk

and Two Penn Plaza, New York, NY 10121-2289, USA

First published 2013

A catalogue record of this book is available from the British Library

ISBN-13: 978-0-33-524418-8 (pb)
ISBN-10: 0-33-524418-1 (pb)
eISBN: 978-0-33-524419-5

Library of Congress Cataloging-in-Publication Data
CIP data applied for

Typesetting and e-book compilations by
RefineCatch Limited, Bungay, Suffolk

Praise for this book

"Such an informative and engaging book, a 'toolkit' for student social workers and practitioners to reflect upon, when dealing with complex cases. This book encompasses in depth discussions, surrounding insightful case studies; which are thought provoking and gives the reader a deeper level of understanding, whilst incorporating significant research, legislation and theoretical frameworks, which underpin good social work practice. An extremely valuable resource for all practitioners!"

Faye Egalton, Student social worker, University of Kent, UK

"This innovative book explores the use of communication through five practice examples. Each practice example utilizes verbatim dialogues between professionals and service users to explore communication. This approach is unique and unlike other books which attempt to explore communication through the use of case studies. There are comments that follow the dialogues to support the understanding of the meaning of the dialogues and offers suggestions for improvements and alternative dialogues. There are good links to theory, methods, values and ethics, research and critical reflection. Both students and qualified social workers will find this book useful in developing, analysing and critically reflecting on their communication skills."

Sally Lunnon, Early Years Graduate and Final Year Social Work Student

To the survivors of child abuse who
have provided the inspiration for
this book.

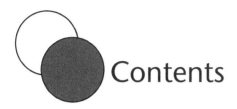 Contents

List of Illustrations   xi

Acknowledgements   xii

Introduction   1

1   **Engagement: Building communication with a young
    person in a context of sexual exploitation**   8

2   **Negotiation: Exploring a multi-agency process to
    assess risk and respond to a child's needs**   43

3   **Investigation: Protecting a baby from neglect and
    physical harm in a context of parental resistance**   78

4   **Use of power: Representing the best interests of
    an unaccompanied asylum seeking young person**   113

5   **Persistence: Overcoming organizational barriers in
    family work with a disabled child**   147

    Conclusion   183
    References   186
    Index   199

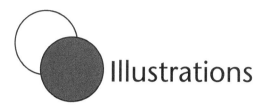

Illustrations

Figures

5.1   Talking Mat   165

Tables

3.1   Johari Window   94
3.2   Child protection case chronology   105
3.3   Incident chart   106

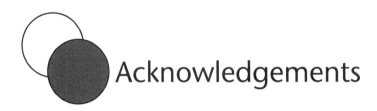# Acknowledgements

We wish to thank Peter McGarry of the Eyewitness Theatre Company for allowing adaptation of two of the scenarios that have been used as the basis for Chapters 1 and 3. The Eyewitness Theatre Company delivers drama-based training modules on all aspects of Safeguarding.

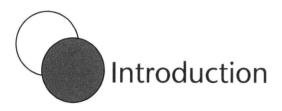 Introduction

Social work as social activism

This book presents communication as central to social work as a profession situated firmly in concepts of human rights and social justice. In the context of extreme cuts to welfare provision and a policy drive to roll back the welfare state and replace it with private provision, it is a tall order indeed to ask the reader to use this book to guide their practice as they strive to retain a firm hold on professional standards and social work principles. Social work happens at the interface of the individual and the state. It provides a buffer zone where the relationship can be defined, explored and challenged. As the book goes to press, social work is in disarray with a new regulatory body, a struggling College of Social Work, government attempts to localize and deregulate statutory guidance and strategies for the wholesale privatization of services. At the same time there is a grassroots resurgence of interest in radical social work and community activism. The Social Work Action Network (SWAN), for instance, provides a focus for a progressive approach which unites service users, social workers, social work students and academics in ongoing debate, campaigning and social action.

The authors attempt to present, based on their practice experience within children's services, real life, current case studies using scripts to illustrate the detail of the work. Five areas of front-line practice are used to highlight contentious areas of social work. These have been chosen to best demonstrate the complexities and nuances of the work in order to emphasize the importance of communication as one component of a highly specialist professional task when located within a politically oppressive climate, particularly for the marginalized. Communication cannot be effective if it is not delivered in a context of understanding the theory and methods of communication, ethics and values and a strong knowledge base related to each case. It is hoped that this book will assist social workers in developing confidence in their skills as authentic social workers competent in resisting all forms of oppression, and acting always in the best interests of service users and the most vulnerable.

Communication as a means of achieving change and confronting misuse of power

It was Friere who stated that 'people are not built in silence, but in word, in work, in action-reflection' (1972: 61). Communication is a form of action. Social workers crucially bear witness to the lives of children and their families and this is indeed a privilege. They do so in a context of social and economic structures that promote inequity and oppression. It is a social work responsibility to promote human rights and social justice when their employers are promoting the interests of the powerful (IFSW 2012). Social work, in representing the interests of children and families, needs to have its basis in good communication skills framed within a concept of social activism. A social worker's lived practice experience must be highly valued because it is formed at the interface of the most vulnerable and the most powerful and carries with it major social responsibilities. Garrett stated that social work is to aid people in communities who feel powerless, 'as the fiery tides of globalisation wash all around them' (2003a: 86, 2003b: 452). Fook wrote about critical social work linking awareness of structural domination with everyday experience and the need to rely on 'communication as a major transformative process' (2002: 18). She stated the need to continually redevelop critical practice so that it is relevant to global and local contexts.

Friere portrayed the role of the *critical witness* as involved in an ongoing process which is not static but active: 'It is a dynamic element which becomes part of the societal context in which it occurred, from that moment it does not cease to affect that context' (1972: 144). However, action must be derived from more than a determination to bear witness. It must also be informed by critical reflection enabling effective action. It is a constant process of reflection on lived experiences leading to the formation and reformation of ideas which become integrated to generate decisions and problem solving and which then feed into new experiences and lead to further reflection and action (Schon 1983).

'When a word is deprived of its dimension of action, reflection automatically suffers as well; and the word is changed into idle chatter – it becomes an empty word' (Friere 1972: 60). Critical reflection, in order to support effective action, must be grounded in a knowledge base and in engagement with dialogue. Knowledge is derived from reference to relevant legal, policy and practice documentation, serious case review material, journal articles, academic texts and media coverage. Knowledge is also acquired through networking with campaign groups, politicians and journalists and consulting with a wide range of professionals, practitioners, survivors, service users, children and their families. Friere also said that without dialogue there is no communication and emphasized that it is an act of creation entered into with humility: 'How can I enter into dialogue if I am closed to and even offended by the contribution of others, at the point of encounter there are neither utter ignoramuses nor perfect sages, there are only those who are attempting together to learn more than they now know' (1972: 63).

Alinsky too wrote of the role of the activist. He spoke of 'seeing injustice and striking at it with a hot passion' (1969: 21) and explored the role of an organizer having 'unreserved confidence in one's ability to do what he believes must be done and accept, without fear or worry, that the odds are always against him . . . He is a doer and does. The thought of copping out never stays with him for more than a fleeting moment; life is action' (Alinsky 1971: 79). Frampton, a careleaver and campaigner, using similar terminology refers to 'warriors for children' fighting a "child protection war" (2009)'. The positive use of conflict is a theme throughout Alinsky's work and he stated that 'conflict is the essential core of a free and open society' (1971: 62). Social work communication in representing the interests of children and families will need to challenge individuals, groups, policies and practices that are detrimental to the safety of children, as well as also confronting the perpetrators of crimes against children. Such a role demands knowledge, courage and persistence. The concept of change and change agents is littered throughout current government documentation. However, it may be the task of a social activist to resist change which poses a threat to the safety of children and adults.

Child abuse is essentially abuse of power and exploitation of the vulnerable by the powerful. Alinsky wrote about 'change coming from power and power coming from organisation. In order to act people must get together' (1971: 113). He described how much of the organizer's work is in painting a tiny leaf but that what keeps him going is 'a vision of a great mural where other artists – organisers – are painting their bits and each piece is essential to the total' (1971: 75). Networking and communicating across agencies and professions is an essential social work skill if children and families are to receive a proportionate and reliable service. This is a challenge when government policies have deprofessionalized many social work and other professional roles and removed some of the systems which enabled good communication to take place. As social activists, social workers need to communicate beyond the immediate boundaries of their workplace because they are professionals over and above being employees. In doing this they need to understand social and political systems and have knowledge of using the media and political processes in order to support the best interests of children and families. Alinsky stated that the organizer's daily work is 'detailed, repetitive and deadly in its monotony', but important nevertheless (1971: 75). Collation of evidence in mapping the detail of cases as a basis for analysis informs effective decision-making and enables the preparation of reliable and valid evidence whether in the context of casework or wider social campaigning.

Integrity, authenticity and accountability

Social workers do not communicate in a vacuum but within frameworks of legislation, guidance and codes of professional practice. An authentic social worker must act with professional integrity. This is generally taken to mean moral integrity and the need to act according to accepted professional guidelines and ethical codes (Banks 2010). Integrity has been recently added as a value and linked to accountability in the International Federation of Social Work's statement of ethical principles – alongside human rights and social justice: 'Social workers should act with integrity. This includes not abusing the relationship of trust with the people using their services, recognising the boundaries between personal and professional life, and not abusing their position for personal benefit or gain. Social workers should be prepared to state the reasons for their decisions based on ethical considerations, and be accountable for their choices and actions' (IFSW 2012). It is also now central to the British Association & Social Workers *Code of Ethics* (BASW 2012a: 2.3) which includes that 'social workers should be prepared to account for and justify their judgments and actions to people who use their services, to employers and to the general public'. These principles are therefore the fundamental underpinning of all forms of communication in social work.

Each social worker in the chapters has a duty of accountability. Accountability 'is literally to be called upon to give an account of what one has done or not done' (Banks 2004: 150). Social workers may be held to account by their employer and the regulatory body which is the Health and Care Professionals Council (HCPC). Social workers have a 'duty of care' to service users. The BASW's *Code of Ethics* (2012a), the HCPC *Standards of Proficiency* and *Standards of Conduct, Performance and Ethics* (2012c) and the College of Social Work *Professional Capability Framework* (2012) all provide comprehensive requirements for social work practice and standards for professional membership and registration.

The *duty of care*, for which social workers are accountable, includes using best evidence and current knowledge to inform practice, drawn from research, policy documents, professional statements of theory and methods, practice experience and service user perspectives. They must understand and weigh up the legal options, powers and duties that apply to specific cases, promote human rights and counteract discrimination, and not accept work beyond their competence. Social workers must also take action when services are inadequate and notify appropriate managers and/or regulatory bodies of concerns that the standards are not being met. These principles are represented throughout the book.

There are often dilemmas for social workers in managing the interface between accountability to an employer and that to a professional organization but the professional standards are clear that the social worker's first loyalty is to the service user. The HCPC states that 'you must act immediately if you become aware of a situation where a service user may be put in danger, and take appropriate action to protect the rights of children and vulnerable adults who are at risk. You must place the safety of service users before any personal or professional loyalties at all times' (2012a). The day-to-day dilemmas faced by social workers who feel constrained by resource-led decisions, for example, must be addressed through competent and sensitive use of communication skills to achieve, as in Chapter 4, an often hard-won outcome.

At a time of severe cuts to services, the BASW conducted a survey of social workers in the UK and concluded that high caseloads, excessive administrative demands, inadequate supervision, high vacancy rates, bullying cultures and low morale were putting service users' lives at risk (BASW 2012b). The lack of safe working environments led Kline and Preston-Shoot (2012) to state that 'greater importance may have been attached to meeting financial and other targets and adhering to agency procedures and customs than to legal and moral duties' (2012: 2). Each script in the book does not therefore shy away from the complex ethical dilemmas that social workers face in contemporary practice.

The BASW *Code of Ethics* states that 'social workers should be prepared to report bad practice using all available channels including complaints procedures and if necessary use public interest disclosure legislation and whistleblowing guidelines' (2012a: 9). The HCPC standards (2012a: 1.11) state the social worker's responsibility to identify concerns about practice and procedures and, with support, begin to find appropriate means of challenge. As in any other situation where the worker is challenging someone who is in a position of power, it is important to gain representation, seek collective action and make use of the organization's protocols.

It is important to understand that social work employers must also be accountable and have responsibility to ensure good communication at all levels of their organization. At a time of increased privatization, when the range of service providers can obscure clarity in lines of responsibility, this is particularly relevant. Employers have a duty of care to the public, service users and staff and must comply with legal and statutory duties relating to human rights, equality and health and safety. The Social Work Reform Board has published *Standards for Employers of Social Workers in England and Supervision Framework* (2011). These employer standards are not enforceable but they should be adopted in all social work settings and provide a basis for discussing issues as they arise.

Structure

Each chapter begins with a script which is divided into a number of dialogues. These tell the story of a social worker in a social work situation related to a child or young person. While the five stories are complex they are not unusual and their content is grounded in everyday contemporary social work experience. Every social work situation is different and therefore this structure accommodates the no-one-size fits all approach to communication with children and young people, their families and carers and the communities, agencies and organizations that surround them. The five chapters of this book trace brief moments within journeys, and the dialogues present snapshots of the lives of children, their families, social workers and other professionals.

The skill of a social worker is to gain confidence in the ability to communicate effectively both as a planned intervention and as an immediate response when unexpected and unpredictable circumstances inevitably arise in practice. Such confidence is derived from lived practice experience, which we cannot provide within this book. The scripts have been selected on the basis of the authors' practice experience and can be used as role plays to facilitate reflection on personal and professional responses, feelings and perceptions. Each chapter centrally includes children's voices because learning is also derived from the experience of children and young people as directly expressed, recorded and researched. All social work takes place in the context of ethical values and standards. Each chapter presents ethical issues relating to the script and although these may be applied across the chapters, the specific topics allow for close scrutiny of ethics in particular circumstances.

Confidence is also derived from a strong knowledge base. Communication will only be effective if the social worker has a deep understanding of the context of their interaction. Each chapter includes relevant knowledge for each specific script. The theories and methods of communication most useful to be applied are explored and interrogated. These are presented in depth with an emphasis on application relevant to effective communication.

However, knowledge needs to include detailed comprehension of the subject relevant to the specific social work referral and intervention, and the chapters address in detail research and academic sources related to each of the scripts. A case study at the end of each chapter provides the reader with a recent real social work situation similar to that outlined in the script, and questions are provided to promote reflection on similarities and differences between the script and the case study. Each chapter concludes with recommended resources and reading material.

1 Engagement: Building communication with a young person in a context of sexual exploitation

Introduction

Chapter content

Engagement at the initial stages of social work communication is often defined as a process which includes an empathetic non-judgemental approach, clear statement and agreement of roles and agendas, fact finding and information gathering and achievement of agreed anti-oppressive outcomes (Woodcock Ross 2011: 18). However, while such concepts may appear obvious and straightforward their application in many social work situations is both problematic and complex.

In this chapter the skills needed by social worker Martin in engaging with Lucy, a young person who is being sexually exploited, are explored from a range of perspectives. This complex social work situation is deliberately chosen because of the need to apply critical thinking to the implementation of accepted social work skills. By unravelling the concept of engagement through a script, the reader is encouraged to explore good practice examples of communication methods and theories as well as an understanding of the extensive knowledge base required in this specific area of work. Also, a contemporary case study is included to illustrate the central importance of social work engagement with young people in the context of serious risk of sexual harm.

Summary of the script

In the first dialogue Maynard, the perpetrator, begins to entrap and isolate Lucy. He uses his power and 'charm' to gain her trust in order to be assured of her involvement with his film project. In the second dialogue Martin, the social worker, feels uncomfortable about Lucy's account of her contact with

Maynard. He starts to engage with her and hopes she will begin to communicate with him about her interest in Maynard's activities. The third dialogue briefly illustrates how Lucy is thinking about her interactions with Maynard as she speaks on the phone to a friend. Further insight is gained during the fourth dialogue where Lucy speaks with her teacher which emphasizes the importance of the social worker communicating with the teacher in order to increase his understanding of Lucy's opinions. In the fifth dialogue Lucy again speaks with Maynard as his influence over her increases. Martin, in the sixth dialogue, tries again to engage with Lucy but instead enters into conflict with her as he lacks understanding of the extent of Maynard's influence. After speaking with his supervisor, in the seventh dialogue, he changes his approach to Lucy and succeeds in engaging with her. This communication provides the basis for Martin to begin his work of providing Lucy with protection from sexual exploitation.

The script: school social worker, Martin, attempts to engage with Lucy whom he suspects is a victim of sexual exploitation

Setting the scene

Lucy, aged 14, is a high achiever and about to take her GCSEs; despite difficult family circumstances she does attend school regularly. Her mother left home recently to live with her boyfriend some distance away, and Lucy's father, struggling to manage, is possibly misusing alcohol. Lucy has been identified by children's services as a child in need. The social worker, based at the school, is just getting to know about her. At this stage Maynard is procuring Lucy over the internet and is grooming her with flattery and promises of a career in the movies, while using some basic Italian to impress her. It is not known whether Maynard is abusing young people himself or making abusive images for profit.

In the first dialogue Lucy is involved in online communication with Maynard. The social worker, Martin, has not yet met Lucy and this communication between Lucy and Maynard is unknown to him. This dialogue takes place in a secret world that Martin will need to discover over time and which will require a high level of skill to unravel. Maynard is always one step ahead of Lucy, pre-empting her thought processes, and he has answers for all her expressed concerns.

First dialogue

Maynard and Lucy chat online.

Maynard: Buon giorno Lucia. Come va? Va bene?

Lucy: Eccellente, grazie. E lei?

Lucy: I got your poem.

Maynard: It's not a poem Lucia. It's a nursery rhyme. A very significant nursery rhyme. Fellini's favourite nursery rhyme. It comes up again and again in his work.

Lucy: Well, I've never heard of it, sorry.

Maynard: Then you know what Lucia, I suggest you find out. There's a rule in movies. If you are going to sing – then sing. No one likes a shy singer.

Lucy: OK.

Maynard: You do want to be involved in this project, don't you?

Lucy: Think so.

Maynard: Oh you think so? We don't sound very keen today do we?

Lucy: I don't know sometimes – it does sound a bit, I don't know.

Maynard: Daunting?

Lucy: Weird?

Maynard: It's far from weird loves, believe me. Innovative. Eccentric. Mind boggling yes. But it's a film about Fellini. Just tell me if I'm wasting my time. I do have other candidates.

Lucy: OK. Don't get ratty.

Maynard: Lucia. I think I'll sign off now. You're having reservations obviously, and I don't need reservations. Been nice chatting to you.

Lucy: No don't go. I'm sorry. Are you there? Mr Maynard. Are you there?

Maynard: Lucia. If you are to get this job I will be your artistic director. As such I will require not only your full co-operation but your respect. Understand?

Lucy: I'm sorry. Of course I want to be involved in the film. It's just that I've never been involved in anything like this. And sure I do have reservations. I'm not sure what I'm getting into.

Comment

In the next part of this dialogue, Maynard continues to allay Lucy's fears. The social worker will need to understand the dynamics used by a perpetrator such as Maynard to entrap a young person into sexual activity that is exploitative. Martin, in order to protect Lucy, will need to understand Maynard's abusive behaviour and how Maynard will use social work terminology in order to reassure Lucy and convince her by sounding authoritative.

Maynard: Then pull out now. But I can assure you you're not getting into anything weird. Let me make that perfectly clear. I'm not trying to seduce you. I'm not trying to groom you. I'm not going to persuade you to meet me. Why would I bother? Even if I had the time. Nothing distasteful loves. I promise.

Lucy: But I really don't know anything about you.

Maynard: What is there to know?

Lucy: I don't know how old you are. You know how old I am. I sent you a photo online and you haven't sent me one. You said your film company had a website but I couldn't access it.

Maynard: I think I want you to do this movie Lucia. You're very beautiful. And I think you have the right skin tone for a black and white movie. And I understand that you're worried. Kids nowadays are paranoid for all the right reasons. There are a lot of weirdos out there.

Lucy: Hey. I'm hardly a kid you know.

Maynard: You will be part of a small, but talented cast, who will learn a number of lines – in your case the nursery rhyme and we'll shoot the whole thing online – using digital cameras, mobiles. Whatever.

Lucy: Yes and then edit it and then enter it into the Cannes film festival next year.

Maynard: Exactly. So what's the problem?

Lucy: Well, why is it such a secret? Why can't it be filmed like other movies in a studio? Mr Deacon says that it will be a technical nightmare . . .

Comment

The introduction of a professional by Lucy into the conversation presents a threat and challenge to Maynard who becomes angry with her. Martin will need to understand that however much Lucy talks with him about her admiration for Maynard and his projects there is always the possibility of an inherent risk of harm which could escalate into violence as Maynard seeks to protect his own interests.

Maynard: Who is Mr Deacon?

Lucy: He's the Performing Arts teacher in my school.

Maynard: This project is top secret. It's art. New Art. I don't want some jumpy little teenager blabbing her mouth off.

Lucy: I wasn't blabbing. It just came up in conversation. I asked Mr Deacon about changing my options to study Performing Arts and it came up in conversation.

Maynard: Don't let it come up in conversation again. Ever.

Lucy: Sorry.

Maynard: You don't seem to understand the opportunity you've got here.

Lucy: I do honestly. I'd love to work in film. I know this is a once in a lifetime opportunity.

Comment

Maynard reinforces his attempt to prevent any contact between Lucy and the social worker and uses his knowledge of an adolescent girl's insecurities. Martin will need to understand that when he first attempts to engage with Lucy she may already be prejudiced against him.

Maynard: The thing about western civilization Lucy is that too many people do not know in which direction they are headed and yet they are all in too much of a hurry to get there. Kids are the same. They are encouraged to get their A levels, go to university and get a degree. No one asks them what they want to with their lives – no one sits them down to discuss it until it's too late, until they find they have to leave university and get a real life job. Like working in marketing or accountancy or being a teacher or a sodding social worker or any other occupation they never really wanted to be.

Lucy: I want to work in movies. More than anything.

Maynard: Going to have a rethink about you Lucy. Need to work with professionals. You've been sounding like a kid who can't handle her hormones let alone a professional arts movie.

Second dialogue

The social worker, Martin, sees Lucy at the bus stop and overhears her chatting with her friends about a film by Fellini. Lucy recognizes Martin as the school social worker. Unusually, Martin gains her attention because he has knowledge about the film that she is now preoccupied with. Her friends tease her about who she was talking about and Martin then joins in.

Comment

In this dialogue Martin is engaging with Lucy in a situation of uncertainty struggling to get alongside her and developing trust. However, he does not have all the information about her situation and misguidedly could reinforce the grooming by replicating aspects of the grooming behaviour by giving her a DVD as a gift, for example. Rather than staying with an intuitive sense of uncertainty to acquire more of the story, he allows himself to be drawn into her illusory world of movies, a fictional world created by Maynard. The centrality of the child is lost to be replaced by a shared interest in Fellini. Martin does know quite a lot about movies because his partner is an actor. He has some understanding about the process of production and is using this knowledge from his personal life to question the authenticity of Lucy's account. He does think that if she has received the lines for the part then the production must be serious but something just doesn't make sense to him. It is a gut feeling that leaves him uncomfortable.

Martin: Federico Fellini the famous Italian film director.
Lucy: You've heard of him?
Martin: Indeed I have. I've got nearly all his movies.
Lucy: Really?
Martin: I'll bring some in. We could all have a look at them.
Lucy: Can I borrow one?
Martin: Sure. I'll bring one in. I'll bring his '8 and a Half'.
Lucy: What's that?
Martin: It's the title of one of his movies.
Lucy: Oh. Yeah. I'd love that.
Martin: I'll bring it next time. You can take it home if you like.
Lucy: I'd rather watch it at school if that's OK. We haven't got a DVD.
Martin: Oh well . . .
Lucy: Yeah, the thing is – Dad pawned it.
Martin: Pawned it.
Lucy: Yeah well he needed the money to pay off a few debts.
Martin: Oh I see. Lucy, are things OK at home. Would you like . . .?
Lucy: No it's OK. My Dad's had a few problems lately. But honest no worries. It's cool.
Martin: You sure?
Lucy: No worries!
Martin: So when did you do this audition?
Lucy: Well it wasn't really an audition. I just sent my photo in and they liked it. They liked it a lot.
Martin: You answered an ad or something?
Lucy: Yeah online.
Martin: So what's the film company? Who's doing it?
Lucy: Capricorn.
Martin: They're quite big aren't they?
Lucy: Are they?
Martin: I'm sure I've heard of them. How did they find you? I never knew you were an actor. Do you have an agent?
Lucy: No. Well. They sort of advertised online. And I sent my picture in. Anyway they were impressed enough to contact me. They said I probably wouldn't need to audition.
Martin: Oh it's just a walk-on then?
Lucy: No. They sent me lines and everything.
Martin: Really? Oh OK. Maybe they want you to read the lines at audition.
Lucy: I have to learn them.
Martin: Oh well you've probably got a good chance.

Lucy: Yeah, suppose so.
Martin: Well done!
Lucy: Thanks.
Martin: Let me know, yeah?
Lucy: No worries. Here's my bus, bye!

Third dialogue

Lucy speaks with her friend Donna on the phone.

Comment

This dialogue is also hidden from the social worker. Martin needs as much information as possible about Lucy's informal friendship networks as her friends can provide an invaluable source of information at the point where the situation escalates into dangerousness. The relevance of Lucy's friendships is illustrated by her conversation with Donna.

Lucy: Hey, Donna, I've been online nearly all morning with Maynard. He's really cool actually – you don't know what you're talkin' about.
He's not a weirdo Donna. He's just eccentric that's all. He's an artist isn't he? I've seen bits of Maynard's movie, the rushes we call them in the trade. He sent me bits of the film he's been workin' on. So no it's not porn, it's art and it's not as if you could recognize anyone that was in them. It was all in black and white and it was very blurred. Well grainy we call it in the trade. It was filmed in Italy Maynard says.
I was talking to Mr Deacon about it . . .
Yeah, yeah, well I'm thinking of changing my options.
Anyway Mr Deacon says you don't shoot a film in sequence. You have to design a storyboard and then edit all the shots afterwards. That's what Maynard says, so he knows what he's doing doesn't he?
Course he's genuine Donna.
No he doesn't even want to know where I live. He says he's not going to meet any member of the cast. That's what makes it so innovative.
Innovative Donna.
You just don't get it. It's like Maynard says, 'Today's morality is just yesterday's prejudice.'
Anyway I gotta go. Here's Dad . . . Dad! He like has no idea. He thinks I still play Mario Brothers.

Fourth dialogue

Lucy discusses schoolwork with her teacher.

Comment

Martin must liaise with other professionals who have contact with Lucy. The teacher's knowledge about Lucy is essential for Martin's understanding of the situation. Lucy repeats Maynard's words to her teacher as a way of testing out the teacher's response. Should this interaction be communicated to Martin, it would assist him in accessing Maynard's methods of abuse and exploitation.

Teacher: Hello Lucy. Well done! You did very well in your mock exams. Mr Deacon tells me you want to switch to Film Studies and that will mean dropping History – your best subject.

Lucy: It's not all about passing exams is it? Yeah, but I want to do Film Studies. I want to work in the film industry. I've been talking to a few contacts lately and it sounds just the right sort of thing for me.

Teacher: Well I don't know much about the film industry. I'm not sure though if it's a secure career.

Lucy: I don't need security. Too many people in western civilization don't know in which direction they're heading and yet they're all in such a hurry to get there. You have to take risks. I don't want to work in an office.

Teacher: Film Studies is not all about acting.

Lucy: Yeah?

Teacher: Might it not be a good idea to have a long think about all this? You're a dead cert to get A level History and qualifications are important Lucy and . . .

Lucy: Mr Deacon says it shouldn't be a problem. It's the start of the year, isn't it?

Teacher: Have you discussed this with your parents?

Lucy: Yes, my Dad's dead keen.

Teacher: Your mother?

Lucy: My Mum's in Glasgow but we discussed it.

Teacher: Yes but you still see her?

Lucy: Yeah, well I'm supposed to go up once a month. But I don't really get on with her bloke. I speak to her lots on the phone.

Teacher: Did you talk about changing your . . .?

Lucy: Yeah. Like she cares.

Teacher: Why don't you think it over?

Lucy: Can I go now, please Miss? I promised my Dad I'd go to the supermarket on the way home. Then I have to go down to the launderette, the washing machine's broken and we can't afford a new one.

Teacher: We'll talk about this again, Lucy. You are university material – you really are.

Fifth dialogue

Lucy chats online with Maynard.

Comment

Martin needs to understand that while he attempts to engage with Lucy abuse may already be taking place. This awareness must inform his communication skills in making a concerted effort to engage with Lucy. Martin needs to reflect on his doubts and uncertainty. In this dialogue between Lucy and Maynard abuse takes place.

Lucy: Hi?

Maynard: Thought you'd done a runner. Haven't heard from you in ages. We have a problem. Quite a big one.

Lucy: A problem?

Maynard: Looks like we can't cast you after all.

Lucy: Why not?

Maynard: Technical problems really. Nothing personal. I assure you.

Lucy: But I learnt all those lines you sent me. Took me ages to get the pronunciation right.

Maynard: Just one of those things Lucy. Sorry loves, really am. You're very beautiful. You'd have been great.

Lucy: If I send you a picture. I can use my phone.

Maynard: Phone would be too grainy.

Lucy: But you want me to use a phone in the shoot.

Maynard: Hey. I'm trying to convince Mrs Maynard here! I'll need something sharp.

Lucy: I've got a digital camera. Well it's my Dad's.

Maynard: You'll need to put it on autoshoot. This means that . . .

Lucy: Yeah I know how to do that.

Maynard: You need to delete the images once you've sent them to me. Don't want your Dad asking embarrassing . . .

Lucy: Give me some credit.

Maynard: Send me them now. But don't raise your hopes.

Maynard logs off. Lucy bares her shoulder, takes a photograph and downloads image.

Lucy: Well?

Maynard: Sorry, Lucy.

Lucy: What was wrong with it?

Maynard: It's a very prudish inhibited teenage photograph and it's unsuitable. Mrs Maynard will laugh.

Lucy: But . . . I thought you just wanted shoulders.

Maynard: I need to see some skin Lucia. I'm not asking you to expose your breasts. But the shot you sent me – well, it's ridiculous.

Lucy: I'll send you another, hold on it's not easy you know.

Maynard: No Lucy. It doesn't matter.

Lucy: Please. I'll send you another. Please.

Maynard: Lucy. I'm really busy.

Lucy: Please. It'll take ten seconds.

Lucy bares her shoulder, takes another photograph and downloads the image.

Maynard: Quite good Lucy. I wonder just a little lower.

Lucy: God, that was low enough.

Maynard: Another inch. Let me persuade Mrs Maynard I've got an artist prepared to go the extra yard. As low as you can go without offending decency. That's what they say in the trade.

Lucy bares her shoulder, lowers her top and takes yet another photograph and downloads the image.

Lucy: Well . . . are you there?

Maynard: I'm here. Mrs Maynard is here too. We can go to the Cannes festival with this one I am certain of that. Ciaou.

Lucy: OK.

Alternative dialogues

In the next section two alternative dialogues are explored between Martin and Lucy in order to demonstrate the dynamics of communication for engagement. In the sixth dialogue (A) Martin endangers his relationship with Lucy through poor communication practice. In the seventh dialogue this is discussed in supervision with his manager. The sixth dialogue (B) provides an example of good communication in this case. When reading these scripts consider Martin's perspective on:

- Lucy's preoccupation with movies.
- Lucy's uncertainty about Maynard's demands.

- The importance of liaison with the teacher.
- The barriers to risk identification and analysis.
- Lucy's family circumstances.

Sixth dialogue (A)

Lucy: Have you heard about Fellini's movies?

Martin: I've seen most of them. They're really for adults to watch not for young people. Come by tomorrow and see me at school and I'll tell you some more about his work.

Lucy: OK.

Next morning.

Lucy: Hi there . . . So what do you know about Fellini? Have you got the DVD?

Martin: Fellini – we'll chat about that later. Lucy the main reason I wanted to see you is because the teachers have been telling me you haven't been doing your schoolwork. They tell me you are obsessed with the internet.

Lucy: I don't need to take exams now I've got this movie part. They're a complete waste of my time and talent. Exams are holding me back. The teachers just have no idea what I want to do.

Martin: Lucy – you live in an unreal world. You need your GCSEs and this internet stuff is just make believe.

Lucy: You just don't know how important it is to me. I'm going to make money out of this . . . Your idea is for me to work in a supermarket and be bored out of my mind. Well I can do much better than that and I don't need any help.

Martin: You just can't see the dangers. I didn't think you were so naive. I thought you were smart.

Lucy: You sound just like my teacher. I'm sick of you going on and on at me. No one believes in me and what I can do . . . only Maynard. He really understands . . .

Lucy leaves and slams the door.

Comment

In this scenario Martin immediately enters into conflict with Lucy who perceives quickly that his purpose in bringing her into the office was not to give her a DVD but to extract information from her about Maynard. She feels tricked. She becomes defensive and the conversation soon escalates into further confrontation until the point when she can take no more criticism and she leaves the room. The social worker has lost Lucy's confidence and this leaves her less protected as she will be unlikely to return to him for further advice, or when the situation becomes too difficult for her to manage. Martin thinks that Lucy is acting as if she is much older than 14 and is manipulating him to get the DVD. Because of his poor communication, he will not get the appropriate information and detail to give to the police and other agencies in order to identify what is known about the film company and Maynard. If Martin visits Lucy's father, this will now be in the context of a conflictual relationship with Lucy and it will be difficult to retrieve the positive communication between them in order to understand what is happening for her at home. Lucy will perceive Martin as forming an alliance with her father against her instead of seeing him as supportive.

Martin is not recognizing the indicators of harm that Lucy is demonstrating. Her body language and conversation content are being interpreted as barriers to communication and he has now pathologized her, even though he is genuinely concerned about the risk. His perspective is informed by stereotypes of adolescents as being difficult to communicate with. Lucy has been defined as responsible for the problem and therefore the solution. Martin considers Lucy as both manipulative and beyond parental control rather than at risk of online abuse and possible sexual exploitation. The focus of social work planning shifts to Lucy's home situation and her father, therefore away from risk of harm from the online abuse. The opportunity to gain more information about Maynard and the risks posed by him are lost. In refusing to bring in the DVD, Martin loses an opportunity to engage with Lucy. He could have managed the DVD material to explore the issues with her as long as he was open with his supervisor about what he was doing and made a clear record of the rationale for giving a gift to Lucy.

Seventh dialogue

Martin speaks with his supervisor following the sixth dialogue (A).

Comment

In the following script Martin gets advice from his supervisor which leads him to revisit his attitude towards Lucy and interventions.

Martin: I've just had a very difficult talk with Lucy. I heard her chatting at the bus stop yesterday with her friend and asked her to come in. She's completely caught up with movies. She sees herself as a bit of a film star and though I've no doubt she's talented, she's not in touch with the real world. I can't get her to take her home circumstances seriously. She's just not listening to me.

Supervisor: Why do you think that is Martin? She seems like a bright enough girl to me.

Martin: Well, she is but she idolizes this guy Maynard who she's been talking to online about films.

Supervisor: Yes, I read your report and it worries me that we seem to know very little about Maynard, and my concern is that your approach seems to be driving Lucy away even though you think she is at risk.

Martin: But this isn't the problem. The problem is that Lucy's home situation is neglectful and her father is doing nothing to manage her behaviour or support her schoolwork. If he was aware of all this internet movie stuff – he'd soon put an end to it. I know he has strong views. I think that I should visit her father with Lucy present and discuss his responsibility towards her.

Supervisor: You're right to be working with family issues, but are you not missing something here? Are you in danger of isolating Lucy and expecting too much from her father? In order to assess the risk, you need to maintain a good relationship with her. Her trust in you is essential to find out more about Maynard and what he's up to. The local child protection procedures are very clear that even at this early stage of suspicion we have a duty to begin a Section 47 enquiry and contact the police. This form of abuse rarely involves one child only and we also need to know if the school has concerns about any other children and the internet. These are the professionals you need to invite to the strategy meeting . . .

Sixth dialogue (B)

Martin speaks with Lucy.

Lucy: You've heard of him?

Martin: Yes of course Lucy, his films are wonderful. I've got some of them on DVD. Come and see me tomorrow in the morning break. I'd like to hear more about the film and your acting.

Lucy: OK.

Next morning.

Lucy: Hi there . . . So what do you know about Fellini?

Martin: The films are mainly about adult sexual relationships. Did you know how adult these films are?

Lucy: I'm not worried about that. I wasn't born yesterday you know.

Martin: It's worth you finding out a bit more about what they want you to do. Tell me something about the company and have you got their phone number?

Lucy: I don't know where they are but they're called Capricorn. I think they are well known. Maynard says I don't need to know their phone number because he can always catch me online.

Martin: Capricorn, they are quite a famous company. Are you aware of safe surfing? Have you heard of the ThinkUKnow website and the guide to how to be safe online? There are lots of genuine people out there, I know that, but also some are keen to exploit young people. You do have to be careful.

Lucy: I know all that – but Maynard really wants to help me get on. He says I've got real talent and I really want to get out of this place.

Martin: Usually, Lucy, genuine people would ask about your legal age and whether your parents approve and they'd talk about contracts and payment. But if you are sure they are OK then what about your friends – would they be interested? What does Donna think? She's your friend isn't she?

Lucy: I think Donna's a bit jealous. She keeps saying Maynard is a weirdo. She just doesn't understand Fellini.

Martin: Well, the important thing is that you are sure you are keeping yourself safe. Think about what you would do if they wanted you to do something that made you feel uncomfortable and think about who might be looking at this performance. Let me know when the audition comes about. Keep me posted Lucy as I am interested. I want to make sure you are OK. You know I will look into how you can develop your acting interests and maybe there are some amateur companies locally. I will see if there are any auditions going on. I can bring in a Fellini DVD and we can look at some of it and talk it through if you like.

Lucy: Thanks, I would like that. Can I come back on Thursday?

Martin: Yes of course. I would like to call in on your Dad too. You said he had some problems with money. Maybe I can help him sort a few things out.

Lucy: OK but don't tell him about Maynard, he'd go mad. He just wouldn't understand. At least you've heard of Fellini – he only knows about Eastenders!

Martin: He is your Dad Lucy. Let's talk more about that on Thursday and why it worries you so much.

Comment

In this scenario, Martin tries to empower Lucy to be sensible and to see the risks for herself and yet he does not wish to alienate her. He does not criticize but is critical of her behaviour because of the possible risks. He makes every effort to retain contact with her and yet plants seeds in her thinking that there may be another less wholesome reason for Maynard's involvement. He also tries to access any information or clues, such as the name of the film company, which will enable the police to make some checks. He has gained information about her friend Donna's perspective and this will enable him to speak with Donna and make some further enquiries.

On Thursday he will seek Lucy's agreement to visit her at home with her father. He wants to see what is taking place at home and the reasons why Lucy is so craving of Maynard's attention. He aims for Lucy to define his involvement as supportive and to help her gain her father's positive interest in her well-being. He uses the offer of a Fellini DVD to retain her interest but also to enable him to supervise her access to the material and inform her about it. This will provide the basis for further debate of the issues with her. After seeing Lucy, he will speak with his manager about the need for child protection procedures.

Communication: theory

Intuition and analysis

Social work decisions should not be judged solely by their outcomes as 'fallibility is an inevitable aspect of the work. They should be judged on the way that they were reached. Professionals need to be able to demonstrate that their decision, however well or badly it turns out in the future, was well reasoned and defensible' (Munro 2003: 110). Informed by knowledge and experience, Martin may have a clear perspective about the risk to Lucy, but implementing his strategy to protect her is a complex and specialist task. Martin is situated between having information and acting. The space in between involves the role of a social worker in making judgements.

When Martin first overhears Lucy speaking to her friends at the bus stop he has a gut feeling, a hunch, that he needs to explore the online activity with her further. Munro referred to this as intuition and it being an essential aspect of the process of making judgements in social work and guiding good practice. Intuition helps social workers to make sense of their observations. When speaking with Lucy, Martin needs the skills to respond and communicate instantly which is a competence derived from practice experience, a knowledge base and an ability to manage and see the relevance of his emotional responses.

Munro explored the balance of intuition and analysis in social work and the use of self as an important social work concept. Intuition 'enables people to draw a conclusion from a vast range of variables almost instantly . . . it draws on people's background knowledge that has been built up over a lifetime' and is 'the backbone of people's ways of making sense of the world and each other' (Munro 2003: 19–20). Schon wrote about the use of 'artistic intuitive processes which practitioners bring to the situation of uncertainty, instability, uniqueness and value conflict' (Schon 1983: 42), a theme also explored by England (1986). Judgements and hypotheses formed as a result of intuition must be tested through collation and analysis of evidence (Munro 2003: 23). Martin needs the skills of a detective in gathering information and being able to critically reflect on his response to Lucy and to re-evaluate this response over time. He must be proactive and not passively await a referral or incident. Knowing how to apply analysis to collected evidence requires the use, once again, of intuition and the mere collation of facts and information will be of no use without an intuitive steer from the professionals involved as to how to make these relevant to protective action. Social work is an ongoing analytical process that involves checking intuitive insights and either dismissing or reinforcing them in order to build further knowledge to inform future action. This is the concept of an experiential cycle explored by Taylor (2006: 191) who emphasized the importance of practice wisdom: 'practitioners are thus involved in creating knowledge about practice through experience rather than simply applying ready-made knowledge to practice'.

Ideal Speech Situation

Martin is beginning to confront a situation of power that is the power of the abuser versus the power of the protector. Habermas referred to an ideal of communication fairness where power dynamics do not distort the dialogue. He called this the *Ideal Speech Situation*. If a dialogue is to be fair then 'all involved must be allowed to speak, all must be listened to and all must be allowed to question others' (Habermas 1976, cited in Blaug 1995: 431). Lucy will be limited in her ability to speak because of the impact of the abuse. Martin needs an understanding of the power dynamics in order to counteract Maynard's power base which remains invisible to the social worker and part of the hidden world of the sexual exploitation of children. Maynard's power is probably based in a network of organized crime making profit from selling abusive images of vulnerable children.

Communication can become distorted because of external constraints such as the pressure of time, lack of resources, managerialism and the social worker's lack of experience, skill and knowledge. When social workers deal with contentious issues, there can be communication distortion because of the power of the agency and the impact of policy directives. Habermas referred to pressure tactics being used, information becoming withheld and the ideal speech situation becoming lost to one that is 'power saturated' (1976). Martin may find himself having to comply with a procedural based, time limited, tick-box approach to Lucy's situation which interferes with his slowly developing mutual trust with Lucy and his creative, situated judgement about intervention.

The social work relationship which was the central tool of social work practice has, in this century, been subsumed as technology became the primary agent of change, permeated every aspect of the social work role and 'stripped the social work relationship of its social, cultural and professional significance' (Parton 2008: 260). Parton also commented that discretionary decision-making by front-line practitioners increasingly became secondary to compliance with prescribed, detailed procedural guidance. Knowledge became relevant only insofar as it assisted the gathering, assessing and monitoring of information which became the central focus of the work and information became the property of managers not practitioners. The focus shifted from observing, understanding and explaining the causes of behaviour to reacting to the results of that behaviour. Howe (1996) described this as a shift from in-depth explanations which were replaced by surface considerations. The emphasis was on systems being in place which provided standardized, easily managed services. However, Carol Smith argued that in social work such certainty is not possible, and that the changes substituted confidence in systems for trust in individual professionals. In order to impose the systems in a situation of uncertainty, coercion is used to ensure compliance. Trust implies, she says, a kind of personal engagement on the basis of which we believe that others will not let us down and involves one person being open with another (Smith 2001, 2004).

If Martin has to complete an assessment of Lucy's needs within a fixed short timescale and produce 'surface' outcomes which do not include assessment of underlying causes of the observed behaviours, such as her behaviour at school and involvement in school work, he may well fail in this task. Lucy would risk being defined as non-compliant and Martin's case might be closed at the end of an assessment time frame. Lucy would be like one of the young women in Nelson's research who said: 'I just stopped going, you know? I'm not sure they even noticed. They didn't care probably, because I was such a problem' (Nelson 2007: 35).

The process, guided by operational targets, would lack meaning in relation to Martin's careful, sensitive development of a social work relationship of trust with Lucy which cannot be time limited if it is to proceed at the young person's pace. A police detective would not be required to solve a crime within a fixed span of time and Martin is needing to use investigative skills in working with a situation probably involving organized crime. He will need to assist police in targeting Maynard by gathering intelligence that can inform their investigation, such as the name of the film company. He will constantly assess the risk to Lucy over time and the need for intervention. Ferguson wrote of social work being complex and not reducible to a set of protocols. He discussed concepts of place as well as time: 'Without movement, someone getting up from their desk, leaving the office and doing something, there is no protection' (Ferguson 2004: 15). Yet social workers currently spend up to 80 per cent of their time at computers inputting data (White 2008). Martin, in relating to Lucy, whose life is unpredictable and uncertain with the strings being pulled by a perpetrator, must reach out to her and find places to meet where she feels comfortable at times she can manage. Nelson reports the young people as wanting neutral venues such as young people's organizations rather than school or home (Nelson 2007: 31).

Communication: methods

Use of trust and authenticity

Maynard is an expert at developing a trusting relationship with Lucy in order to persuade her to become compliant with his orders. It is important for Martin to know this so that he does not unwittingly compete with the grooming methods which perpetrators will go to in entrapping a young person into their abusive network offering, for example, inducements and bribes. Martin will instead offer an authentic relationship (further discussed in Chapter 3) and endeavour to build up trust with Lucy to counteract the contact she has with Maynard, providing a basis for seeing her with her father and exploring her relationship with her absent mother. He needs her to engage with him in planning a safe future career and in being a bridge for her between himself and other professionals who can help to protect her or respond to her needs. Nelson's research of young people's views following sexual abuse informs us of what they most value in contact with social workers. A pressurized approach is not appropriate for a young person already experiencing pressure from the abuser: 'We don't want "come on, I know someone's abusing you, I know they are, who is it?".' One young person appreciated a social worker who 'didn't judge me, she understood the kinds of ways I would feel without me telling her . . . and gave me space even when my behaviour must have seemed weird and didn't make sense – even to me'; 'the adults praised were honest, thoughtful, empathetic, kind and imaginative in trying to make difficult and humiliating situations easier for children' (Nelson 2007: 38). Lucy is vulnerable to Maynard's approaches which will breach the boundaries of acceptable adult/child relationships. The social worker role is to offer a caring relationship within clear boundaries. This involves the 'use of self' and demands emotional awareness, flexibility, creativity and consistency (Lefevre 2010: 33).

Nelson says that children will know which social workers can or cannot hear the young person (Nelson 2007: 25). 'Children are often too powerless, traumatized, confused or frightened to speak directly and may also lack the conceptual understanding or vocabulary to do so. Instead they expect that trained professionals should be able to pick up on emotions and things that are left unsaid. It is in such ways that practitioners should be able to hear children's concerns and act upon them accordingly' (Lefevre 2010: 36).

Nelson cited a young person who said that 'staff need to ask direct questions instead of tiptoeing around kids like eggshells. They must look confident to the kids who are already feeling disgusted and ashamed at themselves. They should be more specific when asking a child, because children don't know how to say it' (2007).

This is exactly what Martin needs to do to use his knowledge base and intuition to make a judgement about what Lucy is *not* saying and to make an assessment of why this is the case. He needs to be confident in his assessment and constantly prepared to revise his thinking given new information and circumstances. He is faced with gaps in knowledge and has to form working hypotheses about what information is missing and then test these out against his background of expertise and advice sought from managers and specialist agencies.

Martin establishes boundaries when he suggests speaking with Lucy at his office and when he begins to point her in the direction of safe activities which interest her. Offering Lucy a DVD is not wrong in itself but needed to be in a safe context and as a shared interest. It might help Martin to get alongside Lucy and to build a trusting relationship, but would be useful only when contained, (for example, Lucy would need to return it within a timescale and Martin would need to inform his supervisor and make a record of what he had given to her and why. The DVD could then form the basis of further discussion about the content and lead to Lucy opening up more about her contact with Maynard, her hopes and aspirations.

Maynard exerts power over Lucy and has an awareness of her vulnerability and needs and he also becomes quite intimidating towards her. When Lucy is frightened of Maynard and has become so entrenched in the activities that it is difficult for her to pull out, Martin needs to assert his own authority by convincing Lucy that he also has a power structure to combat that of the abuse network. Thorpe (2011) in examining notions of power emphasized the importance of social workers using their 'power to' and 'power with' service users in order to achieve positive change. Social workers, critical of their authoritative role, have been preoccupied with 'power over' and consequently have insufficiently used their power as a means of confronting oppression (Okitikpi 2011: 85). This concept is explored further in Chapter 4. At the engagement stage of the work Martin can provide Lucy with knowledge about how his, and other agencies, work together to protect children from harm. This will provide her with the opportunity to escape Maynard's abusive activities when she is ready to do so and has the courage to acknowledge the risk involved. Child abuse is essentially abuse of power and exploitation of the vulnerable by the powerful. Bourdieu's concept of 'cultural capital' is helpful in understanding that certain people, depending on their position of power and status, will have greater cultural resources to draw on in terms of influencing others and exercising power (Bourdieu cited in Thompson 2011: 25). Martin can discover his own 'cultural capital' as a social worker. He can proactively implement child protection protocols working within a framework with other professionals to collate important information and to devise a protection plan. This would enable him to protect Lucy and confront Maynard.

Communication: ethics and values

Children's rights

Social work knowledge comes alive in a context of ethics and values. Underpinning Martin's knowledge base about the use of abusive images in the exploitation of children must be his determination to challenge childism which is the oppression of children and denial of their rights. Lucy has a legal right to protection from harm (Children Act 1989; United Nations 1989: Articles 19, 34). The Children Act 1989 includes the principle that the best interests of the child must be the main consideration at all times (Children Act 1989; United Nations 1989: Article 3). The legislation also requires social workers to respect the wishes and feelings of young people bearing in mind their age and understanding. Martin will need to engage with Lucy so that she will allow him to support her in escaping entrapment by Maynard. If Lucy continues to wish to be in contact with Maynard then Martin will need to consider how he can represent her best interests as these are clearly in conflict with and must take precedence over compliance with her wishes and feelings.

Martin also has a duty to seek justice for children. Martin will work with Lucy openly and yet may also need to work discreetly with a police operation to target Maynard's activities. Social workers working within Section 47 (Children Act 1989) protocols may find that their methods of working need to be hidden from the young person to protect intelligence, and this may appear somehow secretive. Lucy's best interests in achieving justice will be met if sufficient evidence is properly collated to enable a prosecution to take place. This approach will protect not only Lucy but other children. While such action is progressing over time, Martin may need to be selective in his communication with Lucy and her family in order not to undermine a police investigation.

Martin's prime professional responsibility is to Lucy. He needs support to keep the case open over time and sustain regular contact with her, complete the multi-agency protection plan, have good quality, regular supervision, a reasonable caseload and specialist training. If Martin finds that he cannot implement a protection plan for Lucy, despite speaking to managers about it, then he will need to consider how he takes the matter further. This issue is addressed in Chapter 5 where persistence is explored.

Agency and protection

Professionals committed to empowering young people face dilemmas when required to monitor the sexual activity of vulnerable young people. However, promoting their agency must not be confused with a reluctance to recognize risk, and a resistance to monitoring the predatory and grooming behaviour of those who sexually exploit young people. Social workers need to distinguish between acceptable sexual experimentation between young people and abusive sexual behaviour. The London Child Protection Procedures (LCSB 2010) provides a useful guide when assessing sexual behaviour which may be exploitative.

In Rochdale in 2012, nine men were convicted of sexual crimes against five girls following a police investigation of sexual exploitation named 'Operation Span'. The case of 'Suzie', in an analysis of the multi-agency working, exemplified the legitimacy that social workers attached to the crimes being perpetrated against her: 'social work practitioners and managers wholly overestimated the extent to which Suzie could legally or psychologically consent to the violence perpetrated against her' (RBSCB 2012: 19). Indeed, the report critically refers to Suzie at 16 years old being considered by professionals to be 'making her own choices' (RBSCB 2012: 12).

Communication: knowledge base

Analysis of terminology

'We have very little knowledge about the children who appear in child pornography – very few are ever identified' (Taylor and Quayle 2003: 19).

It is very important for Martin to have a strong knowledge base about online abuse of children, in order to understand what is happening to Lucy, and how he may best communicate with her in order to protect her best interests. With a background knowledge about the extent of this form of abuse Martin will be better able to communicate with Lucy in a wider context of likely or actual harm. First it is important in all aspects of communication to be clear about the terminology used. The language social workers use frames their thinking and many words have become commonplace in minimizing and normalizing crimes against children. Even the word 'abuse' is often used instead of the word' crime' at a stage when the criminal aspect is quite clear and the word 'paedophile' is used instead of 'child sex offender' when the word literally means someone who loves children rather than someone who harms them. This excerpt from an Interpol document explains clearly why the term *child pornography* is no longer acceptable:

A sexual image of a child is 'abuse' or 'exploitation' and should never be described as 'pornography'. Pornography is a term used for adults engaging in consensual sexual acts distributed (mostly) legally to the general public for their sexual pleasure. Child abuse images are not. They involve children who cannot and would not consent and who are victims of a crime.

The child abuse images are documented evidence of a crime, not as police would photograph a crime scene where the crime has already been committed, but as a 'crime in progress' – a child being sexually abused.

The terms 'kiddy porn' and 'child porn' are used by criminals and should not be legitimized although legislation in some countries may use terms like 'child pornography' making the term at times difficult to avoid.

Precise definitions are essential and better and more descriptive definitions of such material are: 'Documented child sexual abuse', 'Child sexual abuse material', 'Child sexual exploitive material', 'Depicted child sexual abuse', 'Child abuse images'.

(Interpol 2011)

Crime and abusive images of children

Social workers often become concerned about over-intervention in families and fear making false assumptions when limited but relevant information comes to their attention. Having a solid knowledge base about the subject strengthens a social worker's confidence in intervention, particularly at an early stage of suspicion or concern of child abuse. With this knowledge base Martin would also feel more able to challenge and accurately inform other professionals about this form of abuse.

Abusive images of children are rarely isolated examples of a few pictures taken by an individual perpetrator. Since the development of a mass international market the images are distributed by networks of organized criminals and the industry is worth more than the drugs industry, with far fewer resources dedicated to the investigation and prosecution of the crime. Child exploitation on the internet ranges from photographs to visual recordings of sexual crimes. Because of the global reach of the internet, the posting of child abuse material online constitutes an international crime requiring an international response. Every abusive image of a child is produced in the context of child exploitation and suffering. The children in the pictures are subjected to degrading and humiliating acts of a criminal nature. In some they are beaten, burnt and are victims of other forms of torture. Sometimes they are made to pose in sexual situations with other children, thus adding to their psychological distress. A high percentage of offenders are known to the child as family members or acquaintances and use abusive images prior to committing sexual crime against the child (Mitchell et al. 2005). Children have a right to be protected from this harm and to gain therapeutic support in healing from the trauma.

Online abuse cannot be separated from offline abuse. In the UK, about eight million children access the internet and 1 in 12 have met someone offline that they initially met online (LSCB 2010: 5.25.15). Once imagery is online, the child has no control over who sees the images and could remain a target for perpetrators who often work within networks. In 1998, police discovered over 200 members of a network named Wonderland. Each member had to submit thousands of new child abuse images to the site. Of the 1263 boy and girl victims, mainly under the age of 10, only 16 were identified. Operation Ore conducted by the US Postal Service exposed a website hosted in Texas which individuals accessed by credit card. This led to 7000 suspects being identified in the UK of whom over 1500 were arrested (NSPCC 2008). Since these investigations, the vast extent of this form of crime has been revealed. The NSPCC (2010) collated news reports about criminal convictions for making, possessing, or distributing indecent images of children and/or child sexual abuse and found that more than two million online images of children were circulated by 100 child sex offenders convicted in a period of 20 months. All but one of the offenders were men, ten per cent had been hoarding images for over five years, a third used peer-to-peer file sharing or distributed the pictures online and one in six had a conviction for sexual assault or grooming a child for sex. Fifty thousand of the images were in the most severe categories of abuse which included showing babies raped by adults. One in four offenders were in a position of trust in relation to the child such as teachers, clergy, doctors, police and social workers.

New technologies are being used to transmit abusive images such as mobile phones, digital cameras and MP4 players, all of which are extremely difficult, if not impossible, to monitor and peer-to-peer software enables people to take files from each other's computers without going via the internet, making it difficult to trace. There is a clear link between accessing child abuse images and contact sexual abuse crimes although this area is under-researched as yet and statistics vary from 15 per cent to 40 per cent.

A Save the Children report, *Visible Evidence – Forgotten Children* (2006), emphasized the difficulty in gaining information about this crime because child sexual abuse is a subject shrouded in secrecy and denial, with the vast majority of abused children and adult survivors remaining silent throughout their lives. It would be extremely unlikely for Lucy to go to a local police station to report her worries about Maynard's activities. Martin must understand the importance of listening to every piece of information Lucy provides, often unwittingly, and he must slowly piece together the evidence and not expect Lucy to speak openly to him about what is happening. Lucy is unlikely to disclose because she does not define what is happening as abuse and does not see herself as a victim of crime or of coercive grooming techniques by Maynard. At a later stage, it could also be because she is afraid of suffering harm from Maynard if she tells and has a sense of shame in relation to her friends and family finding out (Kerrigan Lebloch and King 2006).

Research in Sweden (Svedin and Bach 1997) with a sample of ten child victims of abusive images found that not a single child had told anyone unprompted of the abuse. There were no spontaneous revelations. The children had not told parents, friends, siblings or any other adults just as Lucy, when she becomes more worried, does not tell her best friend Donna, her father or teacher. The abuse is generally exposed when the police identify the images. Internet Watch Foundation (IWF) research, based on 1000 adult users of the internet in 2008, found that only 6 per cent of those exposed to abusive images had reported it to police, 4 per cent to the internet server, 4 per cent to a charity and 11 per cent to a hotline; 47 per cent had ignored it and 30 per cent would have reported it but did not know how to (IWF 2008). Sjoberg and Lindblad (2003) found that the abused children denied or belittled their experiences, that there was an absence of false claims of sexual abuse and that recall was impaired by their attempts to forget the abuse-related memories.

Martin also needs to understand the serious impact of this form of abuse on Lucy and the importance of intervening as soon as possible to protect her. The theory of the *child sexual abuse accommodation syndrome* is relevant here in describing a dynamic of a child abuse disclosure (Summitt 1983). Children are commonly met with denial by those they tell about the abuse which leads to suppression of the information and finally, through pressure and fear, to a retraction of the allegation. When police identify images the evidence is indisputable. The child is confronted with the horror of the disclosure that they have been keeping so secret. The impact of the knowledge that the images have been found is devastating and yet brings a sense of relief and enables protection to take place. The Swedish research discovered that some children could, post disclosure, speak about their experiences without great anxiety, blamed the perpetrator and went on to function well at school and home. Some children avoided the subject because they remained in fear of the perpetrator and retained a sense of shame. Others developed severe post traumatic stress syndrome driven by feelings of blame and shame and were unable to get the events out of their minds. They also displayed over-sexualized behaviour and were at risk of further exploitation. There were some children who identified with the abuser, continued to defend them and repeated their own trauma through sexually approaching other children. Those children who had been exploited for more than a year showed the most concerning responses. Importantly, when the abuse was first disclosed to the children they had a 'great feeling of conspiracy and had little trust in adults. This period was described as traumatic and chaotic.' They were particularly worried about who had seen or recognized the images which caused a severe anxiety state to continue long after the exploitation had ceased. They were also concerned about the images being used to groom other children (Svedin and Bach 1997: 21–23).

The legal context

Article 34 of the Convention on the Rights of the Child (United Nations 1989) declares that governments must undertake to protect the child from all forms of sexual exploitation and sexual abuse. They must take all appropriate measures to prevent the inducement or coercion of a child to engage in any unlawful sexual activity, the exploitative use of children in prostitution or other unlawful sexual practices and the exploitative use of children in pornographic performances and materials.

Martin's knowledge base needs to include an understanding of the risk of the illegal nature of the activities perpetuated by Maynard so that he can liaise with police at an early stage of suspicion. In this scenario Maynard made sure that Lucy took the photographs herself, thus removing him from that role. However, some of the crimes listed below might well have applied in the case of post investigation. Maynard might try and argue that his work is art, a creative work and not abusive. The public debate about what is acceptable in the world of art is constantly changing. Betsy Schneider, whose exhibition included 63 photographs of her 5-year-old daughter naked, was not allowed to exhibit in the UK following public outcry (Tyndale 2004). Where crimes are suspected or known to be committed against children then 'art' is never a defence.

The Protection of Children Act 1978 and the Criminal Justice and Public Order Act 1994 address the possession, making, distribution, showing and advertisement of indecent photographs of children. The word 'indecent' has not been strictly defined but case law states that it is for the jury to decide. An indecent image of a child is a visual record of the sexual abuse of a child, either through sexual acts by adults, other children (or which involves bestiality), or children posed in a sexually provocative way. The 1978 Act covers a wide range of offences concerning indecent photographs of children including the making of 'pseudo-photographs' whether made by computer graphics or otherwise. It is a serious arrestable offence to seek out images of child abuse. The making of (this includes the voluntary down-loading of) and possession of such images carries maximum sentences of ten and five years respectively. There are five levels of offence ranging from one to five which influence sentencing and assess the psychological profile of the offender.

The Sexual Offences Act 2003 includes sections which would have had relevance to Maynard's activities. The Act extended the law to include indecent photographs of children age 16 and 17. It introduced new offences to deal with the exploitation of children through child abuse images, providing protection up to the age of 18. These include causing or inciting child abuse images, controlling a child involved in child abuse images and arranging or facilitating child abuse images. It also introduced a new offence of meeting a child following sexual grooming (Home Office 2004; NSPCC 2008). Grooming includes when an offender seeks to interact with a child under the age of 16, possibly sharing hobbies and interests in an attempt to gain trust in order to prepare them for child sexual abuse.

The intention behind these provisions is to provide maximum protection for children from those who exploit or seek to exploit them for the purposes of sexual exploitation or pornography. As these are very serious offences, the public interest will normally require a prosecution. However, the UK's Child Exploitation Online Protection Centre (CEOP) reported that a central database of abusive images is needed, similar to those established in other European countries, in order to identify the children and that prosecuting those who download the images is not enough. Mick Moran, Head of International Child Protection at Interpol, said we are 'forgetting the fact that each of these images, each of these movies, contains a victim' (Jones 2011).

Proactive child protection intervention and adolescent development

Adolescent identity is defined not just by the confusion and emotional conflict inherent in this developmental life stage but also by the social upheavals and changing contexts that dominate young people's worlds (Taylor 2003; Parrish 2010).

Briggs (2008: 15) described the uncertainties of leaving childhood on the journey towards adulthood, and finding new ways of understanding and negotiating in a different arena: 'This means encountering turbulence in the sociocultural context and the fluctuating, shifting, rapidly changing and uncertain adult world.' Well-adjusted and cared for young people manage this transition and exploration with more or less success depending on variables such a personality type, relationships, and adaptability. Less fortunate adolescents, those whose problematic attachments, difficult or abusive experiences and neglectful carers, when superimposed on a roller-coaster of emotional and identity formulation, are most likely to find themselves the recipients of children's services. While much of the literature on adolescent/adult relationships refers to what Daniel et al. (1999) call the *generation gap*, they advise against an over-statement of this concept as a way of explaining adolescents' difficulty in communicating with adults, particularly parents or carers. They refer to a study (Steinberg 1993, cited in Daniel et al. 1999) whose findings demonstrated that three-quarters of those teenagers interviewed were positively disposed to their parents and the conflicts were more to do with day-to-day concerns of tidiness and parental expectations. Assuming that adolescent service users are inevitably going to present as difficult to engage reinforces an unhelpful stereotype and a negative attitude which perceptive young people pick up and react against.

Notwithstanding the above, however, there is little doubt that when it comes to sexuality the notion of the 'generation gap' holds sway with adolescents relying more on peers than parents for their information, discussions and confusions (Daniel et al. 1999). This aspect of adolescent development is complex and it is imperative for social workers, and in this case Lucy's social worker, to be acutely aware of the developmental factors that are likely to determine her behaviours, responses and communication patterns. To this end, he must formulate a developmentally congruent and enabling communication strategy as a distinct piece of work towards engagement with Lucy. His intuitive uncertainty about Maynard indicates a possible risk but without more information that risk is unlikely to be substantiated and therefore the possibility of leaving Lucy unprotected is very real. The fact that young people find discussion about their developing sexuality with adults difficult is very important here, as Martin must find a non-intrusive way of negotiating through these developmental indicators to have any chance of exposing the potential danger of Maynard (Taylor 2003). Lucy's self-consciousness and low self-esteem must be understood as barriers, otherwise it will be more of a potential coup de grâce for Maynard. This understanding will provide a context within which Martin can set out a sensitive and assertive intervention that is both respectful of Lucy's age and stage while acknowledging her vulnerability and potential risk.

Maynard is carefully setting out to exploit Lucy. It is crucial therefore for professionals working with her to have an awareness of her specific vulnerability to being targeted for sexual exploitation. The experiences of sexually exploited adolescents, some of whose stories have been shared in Taylor-Brown's research (2002), leave us in no doubt as to its impact and implications. Charlotte, as a young person who experienced sexual exploitation, said: 'I was only thirteen and he treated me like a queen. He told me he loved me and he made me depend on him. He made me believe that if he wanted to he could turn the sky black, or he could make the sun shine or he could make it rain, he could do anything for me at all and he made me believe it. I made the mistake of telling him I'd been abused, you know, that things were bad at home and stuff because he like reached into that and he drew it out of me and like pulled on strings' (Taylor-Brown 2002: 2).

Being able to engage and communicate with young people within a context of knowledge, informed judgement and sensitive understanding in this particular area is therefore a core set of professional requirements. The acuity and persistence of the would-be boyfriend, or in Lucy's case Maynard, the perpetrator, must be matched with an accomplished broad skill set and finely tuned communication skills. This complex area of communication and intervention presents a number of challenges for both the young person and the professional, not least the hidden nature of sexual exploitation and the secrecy imposed by the perpetrator. This abuse starts with manipulation towards a sense of complicity and often ends with violence and serious abuse (Melrose and Barrett 2004; Kerrigan Lebloch and King 2006). Sally's account, as another young person who had experienced sexual exploitation, reinforces this point: 'I got left in Epping Forest, hit over the head with a spanner and left in that forest; I had another one rape me as well, that was actually in one of the hotels . . . that messed my head up' (Taylor-Brown 2002: 4). Also, the process of grooming traps the young people, isolating them from friends, family and professionals. Both Lucy's friend Donna and her social worker Martin are in danger of being pushed to the margins.

The ground-breaking work undertaken by Barnardo's in 1995 in The Street and Lanes Project in Bradford and written up by Swann et al. in *Whose Daughter Next?* (1998) has provided us with an excellent model for understanding the process of control which is central to the grooming process. There are four distinct stages: ensnaring; creating dependency; taking control; and total dominance. In the first stage the perpetrator impresses the young person with his maturity and sophistication and he then reinforces this with compliments and gifts. Dependency is created by gradually and insidiously placing himself between her and her friends and family. The declarations at this stage are more persuasive including about love, and sometimes she is given a new name that he says makes her more special to him. Total control soon follows and is attended by a complete erosion of her independence through a combination of violence and threats, interspersed with excessive declarations of need and love. She is now alone and isolated. In the final stage of total dominance he has become indispensable and little she does satisfies him. Her ultimate proof of love and commitment is to have sex with 'his friend' and of course this escalates. In the script, Maynard's 'innovative' knowledge of the film world is used to ensnare Lucy. He reinforces his position by 'privileging' her with his 'celebrity' status and uses technology as a grooming device which becomes his method of abuse. An understanding of these stages is important for the professional who will need to target the presenting vulnerability and risk with the appropriate intervention.

In Lucy's case, while much of her activity will be typical of her generation and time, her family circumstances identify her as vulnerable and in need which is why she has a social worker, and now she is being drawn into Maynard's exploitative plan. It is important for her social worker to exercise again a sound knowledge base in adolescent development that will enable him to interpret the complexities of her emerging psychosocial identity while paying attention to potential risks. Piaget's adolescent development theory of egocentrism can in certain circumstances explain young people's presentation of their experiences which do not reflect their reality. This could be relevant to an understanding of Lucy's vacillation between feelings of utter self-consciousness to a sense of being completely unique (Parrish 2010). Nonetheless, and this is where social workers are required to be highly skilled and intuitive, it is essential that Lucy's conversation about the film and Fellini must not be dismissed as adolescent fantasy underscored by a theoretical perspective.

The Children Abused Through Sexual Exploitation (CATSE) model developed in the London Borough of Camden emphasized close collaboration, trust and good communication between the statutory and voluntary agencies (Camden Area Child Protection Committee 2004; Kerrigan Lebloch and King 2006). As well as identifying and addressing serious risk and abuse, and implementing Section 47 (Children Act 1989), which is the statutory duty to investigate, this model also included a response to vulnerable, targetable children and young people presenting low level risk; that is, combinations of behaviour and presentations which parents or carers may find difficult to manage such as truanting from school, regularly coming home late combined with poor self-image and sexual risk taking. This response was referred to as diversion planning and required plans to be formalized via multi-agency network meetings. This form of early intervention and prevention acknowledged both the vulnerability of young people and the ease with which they can be drawn into networks of abuse. It locates ownership of the intervention in all the agencies (and sometimes families and carers) involved with the young person and placed as central to its success targeted, direct work with the young person (Winter 2011: 20).

Martin, in the first alternative scenario, is using appropriate engagement skills to understand the extent to which Lucy is involved with Maynard. It is also clear that she is not sufficiently aware of how potentially dangerous Maynard is. Given the lack of supervision from Lucy's father, with whom she seems to be having a deteriorating relationship, and her use of adult networking sites she is vulnerable. Martin, while keeping her on side by respecting her interest in acting, and indeed Fellini, must honestly share with Lucy that he is concerned and that he wants to plan a meeting which she will be invited to attend with her father. This is a Network Meeting to formulate a diversion plan. While young people often present as rejecting of adult concern as stated above, it is also the case that they need parents and carers to take control and make decisions when they feel unsafe. It is crucial that they are involved as much as possible. As Eve, a young survivor of sexual exploitation, stated with regard to her dangerous home situation which drove her to the streets: 'I just used to wish someone would take me under their wing. I contacted social services and I tried to get them to help but they just took me straight home. I don't think they really listen anyway' (Taylor-Brown 2002: 17). The Network Meeting convened by children's services would be attended by Lucy's teacher, the school nurse, a careers advisor, her social worker, Lucy and her father. The management of this meeting is crucial to the ongoing support of this family and protection of Lucy and engagement with them must be the focus of the communication.

Meanwhile Martin, under the supervision of his manager, would contact the named police team for advice about the internet site and the 'film company' that Lucy has mentioned to him. The police findings will determine whether the case escalates to a higher risk category and whether a child protection meeting is required. The CATSE model refers to these higher risk meetings as Multi Agency Planning meetings (MAPs). These fulfil the same function as the Section 47 Strategy Meeting (Children Act 1989), as further outlined in Chapter 2, with some crucial differences. *Working Together* guidance (DfE 2010) states that Strategy Meetings are for professionals only. MAPs, however, allow for flexibility about the attendance of non-professionals such as family members if it is agreed by the police that such attendance will not jeopardize a criminal investigation but rather add to the information required. If risk of significant harm is substantiated, a series of MAP meetings and MAP reviews can be arranged, supplementing the process of a child protection conference. MAP meetings formulate support and protection plans while simultaneously gathering evidence against sexual predators and abusers. This must be adaptable to the vagaries of the young person whose lifestyle and risk require creativity and flexibility beyond the demands of prescribed timescales and performance indicators. Should it become clear through investigation that more than one child or more than one adult is involved in the abuse, then it is important to note that organized abuse protocols apply (DfE 2010: 6.10–13).

In cases of child sexual exploitation it is often the family, friends and/or the young person themselves who can provide intelligence towards a criminal investigation. Their support for the plan whether one of diversion or protection is critical because attendance at these meetings emphasizes inclusiveness, respect, the principal of partnership and a shared ownership of the intervention.

CASE STUDY AND REFLECTION

Investigation of a child sexual exploitation network in Derbyshire

In contrast to the fictional script about Lucy, the following case study is an example from practice of a complex social work and police joint investigation into child sexual exploitation. This case study enables the reader to draw parallels with the fictional example and to consider the communication skills which, if applied, could have increased social workers engagement resulting in effective intervention towards safety.

Operation Retriever, in Derbyshire, involved 13 men who were charged with over 70 offences relating to 27 girls. At times over 100 police officers were involved in this investigation of organized crime and 60 girls were interviewed.

A gang of men used drugs, alcohol, trips to the park and rides in flash cars to groom girls between the age of 12 and 18, and verbal abuse was followed by the use of violence to rape and assault them over a two-year period. Girls were picked up outside the school gates as well as other teenagers wandering the streets. The men would get the girls' phone numbers within minutes and then bombard them with text messages. At least 27 girls handed their phone numbers to the men without recognizing the risk. Some were lured because they were already vulnerable due to association with criminal activity. When the men knew the police were investigating, they attempted to silence the girls to prevent them from testifying in court, even offering one girl cash to leave the country. Some girls were locked inside rooms and cars before assaults took place and others were threatened with hammers before being sexually assaulted. After ten months of court hearings nine men were convicted of a range of serious sexual crimes including rape, sexual assault, affray, abduction and sexual activity with a child, as well as causing a young person under 18 years to be involved in abusive images of children. The men exploited girls who were seeking love and support and then raped, abused and intimidated them. Police who worked on Operation Retriever commented that the scale of the criminality was shocking.

The serious case review examined the cases of two girl victims of the gang who were known to a number of agencies where there had been concerns about their welfare over a number of years (Derby Safeguarding Children Board 2010). They were both in care and one lived with foster carers and the other with her grandmother. The agencies involved did not recognize the signs of abuse and the full picture of the girls' circumstances was not understood. Both girls had experienced neglect, significant loss and isolation. They had low self-esteem, little sense of belonging and were confused about their identity. One had a prior history of having been sexually abused. Opportunities for diversion and early protective intervention were missed.

Further to this, there was evidence of significant harm as both girls were engaging in criminal activity, running away, self-harm and drug and alcohol misuse. These indicators were not considered as forms of communication from the young women about what was happening to them. Agencies, acting in isolation, did not know how to respond and none had a complete picture of the circumstances. Separate assessments were made with regard to isolated aspects of the young women's behaviour, e.g. assessments of education, criminality, mental health, employment, general well-being, health and development. Both girls were labelled as 'rebellious' adolescents rather than defined as possible abuse victims and both received criminal convictions for behaviour that should have been dealt with in terms of their status as victims of abuse rather than as offenders. The young women's ability to make informed judgements about their capacity to consent to the abusive activities and their ability to make informed decisions about being involved with the abusers was not understood in terms of their known vulnerabilities.

Various plans, such as child protection, looked after children and youth offending plans were in place but were not integrated. For example, the youth offending plans did not take account of the impact of sexual exploitation. The criminal behaviour should have been recognized as another indicator of abuse and this approach would have influenced prosecution and sentencing.

Neither of the young women were able to speak about what was happening to them because they initially did not define themselves as victims of abuse and also because the abusers were powerful in silencing them. One girl said that she didn't want her family finding out about the violence and was scared to tell anyone anything. One girl told the media that she wanted to escape from the hostel she was living in and the abusers offered her lifts which she defined as an act of friendship. 'With their swagger and charm they wormed their way into my life . . . but their "friendship" was just part of their sick plan . . . I thought they were higher than the police,' she said. 'They made you think they were going to help you. It took a long time to realise what had happened was not my fault and they were the ones in the wrong. I felt guilty as if I had asked for it in some way. But when I look back at the videos of myself during the police interviews I think how I look so young and vulnerable. If I can see that now then they must have been able to see that then . . . There was a big difference between going out with your friends and having a drink and going out with complete strangers. At that time I couldn't tell the difference. The victims of these men are not going to be businesswomen on £50,000 a year because they are not the people that they are looking for . . . They are looking for vulnerable people, the kind of person I was.' She described one of the men as the puppet master – everyone did as he told them to do. She said he was constantly texting her, threatening her and waiting outside her house.

The agencies lacked understanding about the indicators of sexual exploitation and it was assumed that the young women were willing to be with the abusers. They should have been given opportunity to speak about what was happening. The review found that the quality of the assessments was frequently poor with little involvement of the young person, their family and relevant agencies. Such a child-centred approach requires staff to be patient, empathetic and persistent in engaging with the young people. The review concluded that the sexual exploitation of young people had not been on people's radar at the time and to the extent that this was happening had been unimaginable.

'My message to other girls who may be victims would be to remember that it is not your fault and that you should not feel guilty and there are people out there to help. You feel embarassed speaking about what happened but there is nothing to be ashamed of. It could happen to anyone. I was scared the police would laugh at me but I got the complete opposite.' Detective Superintendent Debbie Platt of Derbyshire Constabulary said the convictions had only been secured because of the victims' bravery in agreeing to give evidence. She said that the girls had shown amazing courage and determination to see the men who subjected them to unbelievable cruelty brought to justice. Seven men received lengthy sentences for crimes of rape, false imprisonment, sexual assault and perverting the course of justice.

Informing this section were some articles by Catherine Oakes on www.thisisderbyshire.co.uk website between 25 and 27 November 2009.

Questions to aid reflection

Drawing on the knowledge presented in this chapter, and your learning from analysis of the script, consider the following questions. Consider the manipulation and abuse experienced by the girls in this case and use Lucy's scenario to guide you.

 Consider how a young person's presenting behaviour can be a form of communication which is indicative of risk.

 What essential knowledge would a social worker draw on to inform both an understanding of this complex risk and intervention and a communication strategy to address it?

 In the context of a dynamic abusive process what communication skills would enable a social worker to engage and build trust?

 What theoretical perspectives will inform a thorough understanding in cases of child sexual exploitation, help social workers to make sense of what emerges, ensure a safe outcome for the young people and the prosecution of perpetrators?

Agencies and websites

Social workers need to be informed about the key agencies involved in this area of work so that they know where to access specialist advice and support.

Child Exploitation and Online Protection Centre (CEOP). Delivers a multi-agency service dedicated to building intelligence around the risks of sexual exploitation of children, tracking and bringing offenders to account and working with children and parents to deliver a ThinkuKnow internet safety programme. It has a ChildBase images database which enables checks to be made for prior seized images of a child. www.ceop. police.uk

End Child Prostitution, Child Pornography and the Trafficking of Children for Sexual Purposes (ECPAT). This is an international campaigning organization with publications and website resources. www.ecpat.org.uk

Internet Watch Foundation (IWF). Works to combat online child sexual abuse content in partnership with police, government and the online industry and provides a link for reporting online abuse to the authorities. www.iwf.org.uk

Interpol. Provides a central point of international contact for police. It manages an International Child Sexual Exploitation image database which allows specialized investigators to share data with colleagues across the world and the Virtual Global Taskforce, established in 2003, works internationally to facilitate countries working together to confront this form of crime. www. interpol.int

It Matters to Me. This is an animated child safety DVD presented by Mark Williams-Thomas and Julie Walters. Available from: http://www.youtube. com/watch?v=RPcGSJzf2bU&feature=relmfu.

National Police Intelligence Agency (NPIA). Provides detailed guidance for police about the investigation of child abuse. www.npia.police.uk

Stop It Now. Provides a helpline for offenders and the website has resources to assist professional understanding of this form of crime (Stop It Now 2005). www.stopitnow.org.uk

Recommended reading

Blaug, R. (1995) Distortion of the face to face: communicative reasoning and social work practice, *British Journal of Social Work*. 25: 423–439.

Davidson, J. and Gottschalk, P. (eds) (2011) *Internet Child Abuse: Current Research and Policy*. London: Routledge.

Kerrigan Lebloch, E. and King, S. (2006) Child sexual exploitation: a partnership response and model intervention, *Child Abuse Review*, 15(5): 362–372.

Nelson, S. (2007) *See Us-Hear Us. Schools Working with Sexually Abused Young People*. Dundee: Violence is Preventable.

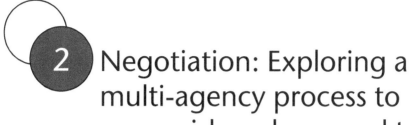

2 Negotiation: Exploring a multi-agency process to assess risk and respond to a child's needs

Introduction

Chapter content

When a group of professionals from different agencies, disciplines and professions explore and debate risk to children, finely tuned communication skills are required to overcome the multitude of potential barriers that obstruct common aims and shared goals. Reaching agreement is central to a coherent plan that aims to protect, and the likelihood for this to be achieved without negotiation is slim. The ability to negotiate presupposes a conducive environment, access to information and a willingness to go beyond one's own perception of the situation in an effort to see the complete picture. Morley (2006: 412) states that 'negotiators must organise a collective process in which they identify issues, develop solutions, choose between alternatives and implement policies'.

The aim of this chapter is to explore negotiation and its place in the communication skill set for social workers through a complex scenario of a child's situation where concerns for safety and well-being cross the spectrum of statutory and voluntary services. This ensures a responsibility for each agency and creates a dynamic for competing agendas and perceptions to be unpicked in order to demonstrate the importance of negotiation in the context of a strategy meeting convened according to statutory guidance. The guidance states:

> Whenever there is reasonable cause to suspect that a child is suffering, or is likely to suffer, significant harm there is to be a strategy discussion involving local authority children's social care, the police, health and other bodies as appropriate in particular any referring agency. The strategy discussion should be convened and

led by local authority children's services and those participating should be sufficiently senior and able, therefore, to contribute to the discussion of available information and to make decisions on behalf of their agencies.

(DfE 2010: 5.56)

The chapter concludes with a summary of the strategy meetings held in the Victoria Climbié case and some findings from the inquiry (Laming 2003).

Summary of the script

The chapter contains four dialogues centred on the struggles of an 8-year-old boy and concerns generated as a consequence of his obesity, his social and emotional world as it is played out in school, and parenting capacity. The first dialogue locates the reader immediately in the world of the child keeping the centrality of children as a priority. The second dialogue introduces the parent in conversation with the head teacher. These participants are also chosen to situate a parent/professional dynamic in an arena that is not singularly social work but demonstrates the significance of the multi-professional shared purpose of safeguarding children. The third dialogue is a strategy meeting where hostile, fractious relations between the attendees provide an opportunity to problematize the process, demonstrating the absence of negotiation and its impact on the outcome. The fourth dialogue provides an alternative strategy meeting that addresses the shortcomings of the first. Through a multi-agency process of negotiation, resulting in an inclusive process of shared aims, this dialogue demonstrates an outcome where the prospects of protecting the child are realizable through ownership of the planned intervention.

The script: professionals communicate through negotiation at a multi-agency strategy meeting to discuss risk to Reece, an 8-year-old boy

Setting the scene

Reece Murray is of dual (African Caribbean/English) heritage and an only child living with his single parent mother Catherine Murray and maternal grandmother Rose Murray. Support from his father is sporadic but nonetheless very important to Reece. Catherine has mild learning difficulties and received Sure Start services in the past when Reece was a baby. She believes she is perfectly well able to take care of Reece – the centre of her world – without the interference of social services. Reece's grandmother feels the family could do with more help but is very sensitive to her daughter's views.

Reece is seriously overweight and both the school nurse and the GP have been attempting to persuade his mother and grandmother to increase his exercise and manage his diet. They accept that he needs to lose weight but Catherine became very angry when on the last visit to the surgery the GP referred to Reece as 'obese'.

First dialogue

Reece has been sent to the head teacher Ms Gayle because he punched another child in the playground and shouted at the teacher who intervened.

Head teacher: Hello Reece. So, what is all this about then?

Reece: [*Looking at the floor, remains silent*]

Head teacher: Come, sit here please! We need to talk about this. We can't have children punching other children. It won't do. It's not how we do things in this school. We respect each other. What's all this about then?

Reece: [*Sits down but remains silent*]

Head teacher: This hasn't happened before. It's not like you. I want to understand Reece but I need to hear from you what happened.

Reece: [*Looks up briefly but puts his head down again quickly and remains silent*].

Head teacher: OK, your teacher told me you just lashed out at Jerome and she couldn't see what the reason was. Was there a reason Reece? There's usually a reason when children do this kind of thing.

Reece: [*Continues looking down*] I don't know.

Head teacher: Reece, please, look at me. I'm going to get to the bottom of this. It is very serious. You could have really hurt Jerome. Did he hurt you?

Reece: [*Nods his head and looks down again*]

Head teacher: Well *he* has no right to hurt you either. What happened in the playground Reece? I'm going to have to contact your mother and I would rather you told me so that . . . .

Reece: No, please don't call my Mum, please.

Head teacher: I might have no choice – I can't wait all day like this.

Reece: He's been saying nasty things about me, calling me names and that. He tells the others to call me names. I hate him. I hate this school. [*Begins to cry which soon turns to sobs but in between manages to speak*]. He says I stink and that I'm fat like a big fat whale. And he calls me Mr Wobble, that there should be a new Mr Men book called Mr Wobble after me. I don't want to come to school anymore!

Head teacher: Thank you for telling me that Reece, I know this is not easy and I promise I will help to sort it out. Jerome should not be saying those cruel things but you must never, ever punch another child. That's not how we behave and it doesn't make the cruel things go away. I am going to speak with your Mum. I know she would not want you to be this angry and unhappy. I'll explain what happened and we'll do our best to work it out. Go and see Ms Ellis (school nurse) now, tell her I sent you to get a drink and I will speak with you again later.

Second dialogue

Head teacher requests to speak to Reece's mother that afternoon when she comes to collect him from school. They are in the head's office and Ms Murray is nervous and unsure.

Head teacher: The reason I wanted to speak to you Ms Murray is because I'm concerned about Reece. He punched another child today during play and hurt . . .

Ms Murray: [*Interrupting*] That doesn't sound like my Reece, more likely the other kid hit him. Why wasn't someone watching them? Reece is a good boy.

Head teacher: Reece became very angry with the other child who called him names and we are addressing this with his parents. But we can't . . .

Ms Murray: That child is a bully and my Reece has every right to defend himself. What did the nasty kid call him? Probably made fun of him being fat.

Head teacher: As I was saying, yes we take this kind of bullying, name calling very seriously and we're addressing it with the children and their parents. But Ms Murray I am becoming quite concerned about a few things. Myself and his class teacher, and the school nurse think Reece is unhappy and punching other children is just his way of showing his feelings to us.

Ms Murray: I don't want my child coming to a school where he's being bullied.

Head teacher: Ms Murray can we talk about why Reece might be unhappy?

Ms Murray: You'd be unhappy if people were calling you names. Reece was just defending himself.

Head teacher: I think Reece is struggling with his weight . . .

Ms Murray: [*Interrupting*] Oh, right, here we go. I knew this would come up. So what if he's a bit heavy. He likes his food, has a good appetite. It would be another story if I wasn't feeding him. Anyway, he makes such a fuss if he doesn't get what he wants.

Head teacher: Ms Murray, we want to help, we can help. I know our school nurse and your GP have been working on a diet and exercises for him and if he . . .

Ms Murray: [*Interrupting, quite angry and raising her voice*] That's it. I've heard enough. Reece is my child and I know what he needs and what he wants. He comes to this school to learn. He gets bullied by nasty kids, and all you can do is lecture me about his diet and stupid exercises. I'm sick of it and I'm not letting him back here again. I'll find another school and I don't want him seeing that school nurse – he hates her.

Head teacher: Ms Murray I know this is difficult but if we work together on this . . .

Ms Murray: Where's my son? I need to get home to get his dinner. [*She leaves . . .*]

It is two weeks later and Reece has not been back to school. Several unsuccessful attempts via letters, phone calls and a visit from the lead professional in the support network for the family, have been made to contact them. A meeting was also convened but Ms Murray did not attend. Concern is growing, particularly in the light of a recent report from the GP about Reece's obesity, worries about attendant cardiac problems and the later development of type two diabetes. All professionals involved have concerns about Reece's low self-esteem, isolation from his peers and a marked deterioration in his schoolwork. The school nurse is worried that he might also be pulling his hair out, having witnessed him tugging at his hair the day he came to see her after punching the other child. She has not had opportunity to check this further as Reece has not been back to school since.

A decision is made to refer to children's services. A social worker, Fiona, takes the telephone referral. A decision is made to undertake an assessment that will include information gathering from all current and previous professionals involved in the case, and, given the seriousness of the referral, an immediate home visit. Fiona is instructed to request to see Reece alone and to speak with him. She is also advised to phone and let the family know she is coming to see them following concerns raised by Reece's school. There is no reply to the call and when Fiona arrives at the family home Ms Murray is abusive, refuses to let her into the house and becomes extremely angry when she requests to see Reece. She slams the door on Fiona who persists and remains outside the home. Fiona phones the family and manages to speak to Reece's grandmother who she persuades to let her in. Outlining her concerns, Fiona establishes that Ms Murray is refusing to allow Reece to school because of the bullying. She also finds out that Reece has not been outside to play for one week, has had very little exercise and that Ms Murray is now antagonistic to all professionals involved. Reece's grandmother seems reluctant to help though she does share some of Fiona's concerns, particularly about Reece's unhappiness.

Fiona reports back to the team manager who decides that there is reason-able cause to suspect that Reece is suffering, or is likely to suffer significant harm. Therefore a Section 47 (Children Act 1989) strategy meeting in compliance with Working Together procedures is required (DfE 2010). This decision is based on concerns for Reece's physical health and emotional welfare which have escalated since the withdrawal of parental engagement and co-operation at this time.

Third dialogue

The strategy meeting is held in the office, chaired by the team manager and attended by the social worker, head teacher, school nurse and a police officer from the Child Abuse Investigation Team (CAIT).

The team manager welcomes the professionals and notes apologies from the GP. The professionals introduce themselves and the meeting commences. The chair outlines the purpose of the meeting, which is to establish, through the sharing of information, whether a child protection investigation should be initiated, including considerations for a criminal investigation, and whether there is a need for any immediate action to protect the child. If an investigation is initiated then the meeting will address how it will be conducted and the roles and tasks for the professionals will be planned and recorded. Finally, a decision will be made as to what information will be shared with the family and this only if it is believed not to compromise either the safety of Reece or any potential criminal investigation.

Head teacher: I'd like to point out please before we start that Sheila (school nurse) and I have been sitting outside since 10 am, when incidentally this meeting was due to start. It is now 10.20 and I will have to leave soon. I have two other very important education meetings scheduled for this morning.

Chair: Apologies for that. We were waiting for the report from the GP that contains much of the substance of the concerns.

Head teacher: Well someone could have come and explained that instead of just leaving us in the chaos of a reception area. Maybe we could have been allowed to sit in here even!

Chair: This team doesn't have control over the reception area. I'm sorry again we were late starting. We're all busy people so let's get on then and hear the social worker's report starting with the child and family details.

Comment

A number of factors can contribute to a negative dynamic limiting the capacity for negotiation and a safe outcome. In this dialogue, the head teacher has introduced a distraction because of her resentment about loss of precious time, and feelings of being disrespected by one of the professionals. This is likely to have a significant impact on how this meeting will progress if not addressed. Thompson refers to 'communicative sensitivity' as the importance of knowing the when as well as the how to communicate (2011:

246). Shannon and Weaver's transmission model of communication also has relevance (1964). They suggested that in the transmission of communication from a source to a destination various forms of *noise* could get in the way and disrupt the receipt of the message. In this dialogue the now emotionally driven hidden agenda has become the *noise* and is interfering with the essential child protection messages being communicated.

> *The social worker provides factual information regarding Reece including full name, date of birth, address, members of the household, ethnicity and religion. She also identifies that Ms Murray has a mild learning disability. A synopsis of the child protection concerns is provided based on the assessments to date. The chair then presents the report from the GP that highlights significant medical concerns for Reece now and in the event that his weight is not more effectively controlled. The report also raises concerns about the ability of Ms Murray to make the necessary links between her management of Reece's diet, exercise and his health.*

Chair: The most pressing concern at this stage would appear to be Reece's deteriorating health and potentially where this will lead without a social services intervention. However, in the absence of the GP it is difficult to determine the timescales and level of immediacy with the health concerns. He also hasn't identified these concerns as risks or stated a child protection view. There is the attendant concern regarding Ms Murray's current relationship with professionals, her understanding of the concerns and the impact of this on any potential for change.

Police officer: I expect if there was any imminent danger the GP would have stated that clearly in his report . . . but I . . .

Head teacher: It shouldn't be for us to speculate. I really think the GP should have attended this meeting but my concern is as much for Reece's emotional and social development and how Ms Murray is clearly not coping. Reece is already being alienated at school and is not reaching his academic potential. I do think however that Ms Murray is doing the best she can in difficult circumstances. She absolutely adores that child and she should have received a lot more support years ago. Children's services must have had knowledge of this family.

Police officer: If I could be allowed to finish please. If this child is suffering significant harm as a result of his diet the GP should have communicated the link. No one here is in a position to interpret medical information [*addresses the school nurse*] – no disrespect to yourself!

Comment

At this point in the dialogue the chair ignores both the substance of the police officer's concerns about the GP and the disrespect to the school nurse.

This serves to perpetuate an uncomfortable atmosphere and uneasy dynamic. The school nurse is likely to feel at best undermined and at worst intimidated. As one of the professionals who has regular and relevant contact with the child, her information and opinion is key to the discussion and outcome. Exaggeration of hierarchy identified as professional dangerousness by Reder et al. (1993) is not an uncommon experience for professionals perceived as lower status to be undervalued in formal decision-making meetings such as this.

Chair: Is Ms Murray receiving any support from the learning disabilities team?

Fiona: No, she's not receiving any additional support at present. But she does have informal support from her mother.

Chair: Right now Reece's grandmother seems not to have the kind of influence we know is required because, if she had, Reece would most likely have been at school last week.

School nurse: I'm very worried about the strain on this child's heart. He struggles to get around and seems to be in a vicious circle now with regard to eating and exercise. I've tried to advise Ms Murray and she does seem receptive when we speak but there isn't any sustained change. Three weeks ago his class teacher observed a few bags of crisps and a variety of chocolate bars in his school bag.

Comment

A psychologist or learning disability expert report on the parental capacity of Ms Murray would have added important information to this meeting. However, because neither the chair nor Fiona have established the parameters of Ms Murray's learning disability, this limits the discussion, not just in relation to Reece's needs but also Ms Murray's right to community-based services and the potential barriers to good practice in cases of parental learning disability (DoH/DfES 2006). McGaw and Newman (2005) offer an assessment tool for parents with learning disabilities. In a specialist parenting assessment manual they advise that assessment should include a range of physical and psychological elements which can affect parenting. This assessment covers cognitive and emotional functioning and focuses in four areas: family history, intellectual functioning, independent living skills; and the need for support and resources. James (2010) draws attention to discrimination experienced by parents with learning disability based on what he refers to as *presumed incompetence*. This can be avoided by ensuring that thorough assessments are made and shared by professionals skilled in this specialist area. James comments that the most common form of abuse by parents with learning disability is neglect.

Police officer: I'm not sure I see a role for us. No crime is being committed here, and really it is a health issue. Has anyone actually sat down with this parent to explain how to help her child to lose weight? Sounds like a family support issue to me.

Head teacher: I'm inclined to agree. I don't think we can get authoritative with a parent who needs support for an identified need and isn't getting it. Isn't the idea supposed to be working in partnership with families? I'm afraid I need to go soon!

Police officer: I don't think it is going to help Reece, going down the child protection path, if all we do is terrify his mother into withdrawing altogether. If every overweight child were to come into this process we would not be able to function.

Comment

Generalizing the issue serves to introduce a more informal discussion, distracts from the specific case and dilutes the risk. A singular perspective in relation to a criminal investigation possibly influences the police officer here. Without the GP present to provide clear medical explanations, concerns for Reece can potentially get lost.

School nurse: But the GP is really worried and if . . .

Head teacher: Then he should be here.

Fiona: He has surgery this morning and could not get away, but he was very clear on the phone when we spoke yesterday that the rapid increase in Reece's weight is likely to put pressure on his entire body, and there's also growing concern for his mobility.

Comment

The GP's attendance is crucial not just because of the nature of the concern and the medical information that needed to be explained and shared, but also the need for shared ownership of the planning and decision-making to secure Reece's safety.

Chair: Time is pressing on and (addressing the head teacher) I know you are anxious to get away. In the first instance we must address the risk to Reece, and whatever the circumstances with Ms Murray. If we believe his obesity will lead to harm or indeed is harming him right now then we need to begin child protection procedures. The GP has been quite detailed in his report and there is also the bullying, self-esteem issues and more broadly his social and emotional development. I suggest we pursue this within child protection procedures and carry out a detailed investigation into Ms Murray's ability to address the weight issues. We can use this time to engage and assess both mother and grandmother and refer Ms Murray to the learning disability team for an assessment and support with our ongoing assessment and investigation.

Comment

The Chair tries to avoid the dynamics by summarizing in a manner that shuts down further discussion, abandons consensus decision making, and is driven more by the time constraints than the purpose of the meeting, which is assessing risk and planning an investigation (Glenny and Roaf 2008). Chairs of strategy meetings must be appropriately experienced, and both skilful and sensitive in their management of the meeting; acknowledging and respecting the diverse professional roles, identities and expertise (DfE 2010).

Police officer: I'm not sure I agree with the decision, as I don't recognize abuse as having taken place, but in any case it would be a single agency investigation and assessment so there's no further role for us.

Comment

This is not an uncommon situation in child protection investigations and is another reason for the chair to be experienced and with sufficient authority to challenge this position. At the heart of good child protection practice there is a commitment to the sharing and discussion of information where 'the role of the police in child protection extends beyond that of only criminal investigation. It embraces other duties and responsibilities, especially as the welfare of the child and his/her needs are the overriding and paramount considerations' (Walke 1993: 194).

Head teacher: I'm also not sure that taking this particular line will help but something definitely needs to be done. I really must go now but you can send me the decisions and actions, or I can pick them up from the school nurse.

Head teacher and police officer leave the meeting.

School nurse: I'm not sure if I should say this because I have no real evidence but I'm worried that Reece may be pulling out his hair. The day he came to my office I noticed him tugging his hair as though it was a response to the situation he was in.

Comment

The school nurse provides some crucial information after key professionals have left the meeting. The information is very important in contributing to the most comprehensive picture of Reece's situation, which in turn is key to professional understanding of Reece and is integral to the decision-making process. White (2008), with reference to the sharing of medical information in the case of Victoria Climbié, provides an insightful analysis into how information is shared and what is understood. Sharing alone is not sufficient in this complex work.

Chair: Thank you. It is very important information.

> Chair concludes by agreeing this plan with the social worker and the school nurse:
>
> • Case is allocated with immediate effect.
> • An immediate referral by the social worker to the learning disability team to carry out a parenting assessment and to support Ms Murray in under-standing the level of risk and working out a strategy to address it.
> • School nurse to formulate a weight reduction and exercise plan with Reece and his family within one week to be monitored both by the GP and the school nurse.
> • Social worker and team manager to undertake a visit to the family home today to discuss with Ms Murray and her mother the multiple concerns for Reece and the risk to his health if the current situation regarding his obesity persists.
> • Social worker, this week, to explain her involvement to Reece, seeking his views about what he thinks might help and work out with him the best way for him to participate.
> • An anti-bullying strategy in respect of Reece to be implemented and moni-tored at school by the head teacher to be in place by the end of the week.
> • Class teacher to monitor all aspects of Reece's education.
> • A date in 15 days' time is set for an initial child protection conference.
> • All professionals to have a copy of this plan.

Alternative dialogue

In the next section the dialogue represents an example of good practice in relation to negotiation and an alternative outcome as a consequence of this. When reading this dialogue consider the following:

- The management of the meeting and the professional atmosphere that prevails.
- The GP's attendance and the impact on the discussion.
- The emphasis on clarity of information and the distinction between fact and opinion.
- How Reece remains central within the context of his family circumstances.
- How consensus is achieved.

Fourth dialogue

The meeting, at the children's services office, is chaired by the team manager and attended by the social worker, head teacher, school nurse, GP and a police officer from the child abuse investigation team (CAIT).

The meeting scheduled for 10.0 am starts on time. The team manager welcomes professionals, thanks them for coming, acknowledging their busy schedules and competing demands, and outlines the purpose and process of the meeting as in the third dialogue. The team manager suggests that the meeting should take approximately one hour and asks if there are any time constraints for attendees. Professionals introduce themselves and the meeting commences.

At the chair's request Fiona presents her report as in the third dialogue. She added that she also contacted the adult learning disability team who have not been involved with this family since Reece was 18 months old when Ms Murray's mother came to live with them. The team did make a referral to the local Sure Start programme and only closed the case once it was confirmed that Ms Murray had started attending. There will now be a thorough assessment.

The police officer confirms that the family is not known to police.

Chair: This is a complex and worrying case where all the agencies involved with Reece and his mother are reporting concerns, but as the referring agency, I'd like to start by taking a report from the school, followed by updates from the GP and school nurse. We will then discuss risk and whether we believe the threshold has been met to proceed with a Section 47 child protection investigation.

Head teacher: The basis of my concern is Reece's presentation in school. He has poor relations with his peers, is socially isolated and he is becoming increasingly aggressive with both children and staff. This is a big change from when he first attended our school. Back then he integrated well generally and had a few close friends, which is not the case now. In my view he was a happy child and I'm inclined to put this deterioration down to his weight gain which seems to have increased rapidly over the past year.

Chair: What about his academic ability and progress?

Head teacher: That's an additional concern. I picked up a report from his class teacher this morning and there has been a marked deterioration there too. Work set is not always completed and his concentration is poor. He is a child of average ability but is not meeting his potential.

Police officer: Is there any possibility that he may also have a learning disability.

Head teacher: Not that we have identified. But it could be that he lacks the stimulation and the supervision he needs with homework. I expect Ms Murray needs more support with Reece and perhaps that's where the problem lies. I'm surprised actually that social services have not had more involvement with this family.

General practitioner: I have known the family for a number of years. Reece and his grandmother came to the surgery ten days ago because he was having stomach pains. His weight had increased significantly since their previous visit and as I stated in my report we are now looking at the medical complications of childhood obesity and potentially very serious health problems for Reece if his weight is not addressed . . . and soon.

Chair: Can you identify for our records please Reece's current health situation and problems you foresee. Timescales for addressing them would be very helpful as this will be critical for our identification of a risk threshold. It is important that we are as clear as possible as to what is evidential or factual at this point, and what is speculative.

General practitioner: The most immediate health problems are pressure to his heart and type two diabetes; we would also be concerned about his mobility. It is difficult to state a timescale but if this pattern is not interrupted we could be in a very serious situation indeed in six to nine months.

Chair: . . . And his mother's response, does she understand how serious this is? How has she demonstrated her understanding?

General practitioner: Ms Murray is very committed to her child and until his weight started to spiral out of control we had a positive relationship with her at the surgery. She attended regularly, asked relevant questions and Reece was doing fine generally. But the school nurse alerted us to worrying weight gain a year ago and since then we have been attempting to engage them in a programme of exercise and diet. No good I'm afraid. We had avoided using the term *obese* until recently as we were afraid it might prompt a disengagement but there was a growing imperative to be medically and diagnostically clear and of course our worst fears were realized. We have not seen Ms Murray or Reece since and that's over two months ago now, except of course when he came with his grandmother. On reflection, perhaps we should have taken advice from the learning disability experts as to how to share our concerns.

Chair: Has she actually missed an appointment?

General practitioner: Yes, she has missed two now, one with myself, and the other with the practice nurse.

Chair: [*Turning to the school nurse*]. Could we take your report please? Your information is key.

School nurse: I've known Reece since he started school. He was never a thin child but really only presented with weight problems in the past 18 months, and recently his weight increase has been so rapid that I thought it was important to discuss with his GP, hence the diet and exercise regime. In the main, and until his weight problems, Reece was a healthy, happy boy and his school attendance was very good. Our relationship with Ms Murray was also positive whenever I had reason to speak to her about Reece. His grandmother has also been very pleasant and quite involved with the family as far as I know.

Chair: What is your view of the current situation?

School nurse: It seems to me that Reece's weight gain is out of control and his family seem unwilling or perhaps unable to help him right now. As well as the health issues identified by the GP I'm also worried that Reece may be pulling his hair out after observing him tugging it quite violently when he was distressed. I haven't had a chance to check this out properly, but I am concerned. I think Ms Murray should be getting support for this from social services. She does have learning difficulties and she has had a good relationship with the school. Maybe she doesn't understand.

Fiona: We have only had one contact with the family and it was very problematic, but there are lots of reasons that could explain it, not least fear of social services removing the child. I am very worried about Ms Murray's withdrawal and keeping Reece in the house and away from school. Rose (grandmother) did speak to me though, and while she wasn't pleased with the visit she wasn't hostile either, probably because she agrees with some of our worries about Reece. She seems very close to both him and his mother. It must be very difficult for her.

Chair: You did get into the house. What observations did you make?

Fiona: Everything looked fine – clean, warm and tidy, and I saw lots of toys and stuff, belonging I suppose to Reece.

Chair: That seems to be all the reports. Is there anything else factual to add at this stage? No! OK, well to summarize: the immediate problem appears to be health concerns regarding Reece's weight and the impact of this both on his education and his social and emotional well-being. Ms Murray's hostility to professionals and concerns for her parenting appear to be recent. Reece's grandmother is an important support for the family, though we don't know how supportive she may be to a professional opinion that may place her in opposition to her daughter. We don't have Reece's views to add, as the social worker did not get to speak with him, but all reports from the school describe him as an unhappy rather isolated child. It is very important that Reece is spoken to by Fiona as soon as possible to make sure his views are central to our assessment and planning.

General practitioner: In my view there is a medical risk to Reece if we can't get him on a healthy diet and an exercise regime, and for this we need to have a co-operative relationship with his mother. It seems to depend on that.

Police officer: I'm not sure there is a role for us here as a crime hasn't been committed but in my view it is a very worrying future for the child if this situation is not interrupted. On the other hand, if every overweight child came into the child protection process we would grind to a halt.

Chair: But he's not just overweight he is clinically obese!

Police officer: All this unhealthy food being pushed at children! Even very with-it parents are struggling to keep their children on healthy diets without having to go to war with them.

Head teacher: In my opinion we need to give Ms Murray more time to understand the importance of diet and exercise. We also need to get Reece back into school and I think we will only antagonize her further if we start talking child protection.

School nurse: I'm not sure Ms Murray fully understands, perhaps she needs more time. It would be so much better if she willingly engaged with us. Our chances of working with Reece would be much better too.

Police officer: It seems to me that this mother has done very well by her child so far, particularly given her limitations – so maybe with the right help she could overcome this problem. With some partnership working!

Chair: Ms Murray's commitment to Reece, evidence of her parenting until this recent concern and the extent to which she has impressed professionals most definitely provide a strong base from which to approach this intervention. It must not distract us from the current risks to Reece. The child is our focus and an engagement with his mother our means to keeping him safe.

Police officer: But will the child protection route enable this engagement?

General practitioner: I'm inclined to agree that Ms Murray's own vulnerability and her efforts until recently are likely to divert our attention and sidetrack the risk to Reece.

Fiona: Perhaps Reece is a challenge to manage around food, and Ms Murray needs to learn parenting strategies. A referral to the adult learning disability team might be appropriate.

Chair: We must establish as a matter of urgency whether or not Ms Murray will engage and work with us. I suspect she is very worried, frightened even; this might take time. The question is what happens to Reece while we are involved in building a working relationship with his mother. His timescales for needing protection are unlikely to be the same as the mother's for developing co-operation.

Head teacher: Of course we must prioritize Reece, but in the longer term and keeping him in mind it might prove to be more sustainable and appropriate to get Ms Murray on board with resources and support. Let's face it, she will need more than she is getting right now anyway.

Fiona: It is the initial social services contact with her that will be most challenging.

Chair: The consensus seems to be to establish a working relationship with Ms Murray and Reece's grandmother within a timescale that reflects the level of concerns and risk to Reece. If this is not achieved, let's say, within ten days – we will have to take the child protection route.

Police officer: That seems reasonable. Reece must return to school and Ms Murray needs to demonstrate that she understands the health risks by engaging with the diet and exercise regime.

Head teacher: I think it is very important that the case remains allocated to a social worker until we are all satisfied that Reece's situation has improved and the change is sustainable.

Chair: We will review the case in ten days and, if progress has been made, a network meeting of all agencies involved can be arranged for three months in order to have time to review progress and consider what is required at that point. If, however, we are not satisfied with the level or quality of the engagement, a child protection conference will be arranged 15 days from then. Shall we put that provisional date in our diaries today? Is everybody satisfied with that decision before we draw up a plan?

Comment

All attendees agree with the decision and the plan, which is the same as at third dialogue except, crucially, that a child protection conference will be delayed to provide opportunity to engage and work with Reece's family.

Communication: theory

Emotional intelligence and reflective function in inter-professional communication

Acknowledging risk of significant harm to Reece by convening a strategy meeting is one of the important early steps on the journey to addressing his safety. The information that will be shared, the professionals attending, the environment, venue and overall context are crucial components of the process in terms of their individual and collective influence. However, it is the dynamic relationships between and among the attendees that will be likely to have an over-and-above determining impact on the outcome. The quality of the negotiation in the meeting is predicated on the ability of the professionals to communicate with respect, care, curiosity and a degree of uncertainty that allows for a rich discussion and reflective analysis.

Awareness, insightfulness, perceptiveness and responsiveness are key to the professional exchange if complex situations such as Reece's are to be understood and progressed. However, this is not easily arrived at. Clear and effective communication can be hampered in child protection fora, not least because the nature of the information discussed can trigger participants to revert to responses and behaviours reflective of their own emotional past. Stress too heightens defensiveness and limits an appreciation of the other. The head teacher, in the third dialogue, feels disrespected by being left waiting in the reception area. She believes that her social work colleagues do not have regard for her time. Powerful feelings of resentment and hostility influence the nature of her participation and ultimately the outcome of the meeting. The social work manager who chairs the meeting feels challenged and uncomfortable and shows little insight into the strength of view being expressed. She is not perceptive to the emotional content in what is being said and consequently loses control over the impact it subsequently has on the outcome of the meeting.

Given the level of emotional content, and the importance of feeling and intuition in the child protection process, it is important to examine multi-agency negotiation from a psychological perspective by exploring the theoretical framework of emotional intelligence (Goleman 1996; Morrison 2007; Howe 2009), and reflective function (Fonagy and Target 1997; Walker 2006). Within that context the following questions are pertinent: What enables the negotiation that takes place in the (fourth dialogue) strategy meeting that arrived at the preferred outcome? What transcends environment, time constraints, and distinct professional knowledge and agency agendas to allow for open dialogue that is at once respectful and challenging?

A promptly held meeting is a very important communication of respect to participants in itself. However, circumstances such as poor punctuality and delay are often unavoidable and generally not the specific responsibility of one individual, but they must be handled appropriately to avoid becoming the vehicle for unrelated emotions and for distracting from the protection of the child. Walker comments that 'inter agency communication can quickly become competitive and rivalrous in which narrow, entrenched positions are taken. In so doing it can become hard to listen and understand the perspective of the other' (2006: 13).

Reflective function for the purpose of communication in child protection, according to Walker (2006), is the ability to understand and relate flexibly to the thoughts and feelings as well as the experience of others. According to Fonagy and Target: 'reflective function is the developmental acquisition that permits the child to respond not only to other people's behaviour, but to his conception of their beliefs, feelings, hopes, pretences, plans' (1997: 679). The extent to which the child accomplishes this capacity can in part be traced back to secure attachment with their primary caregiver enabling confidence later on to question, challenge and negotiate while feeling safe to do so.

For the purpose of communication and negotiation in strategy meetings, it is clear that good reflective function is required to deal with both the overt and hidden agendas that are brought into the room. The police officer in the third dialogue offers a view about overweight children generally. He does not acknowledge the situation as abusive and is dismissive of the notion that obesity in this situation could equate with significant harm. His reflective function is limited in this situation and does not account for the experience of the school nurse whose regular contact with Reece and relationship with him has an emotional base. She is left experiencing his comment as hurtful and professionally insulting. Reflective function 'includes the ability to recognise that other people's behaviour may be driven by desires and beliefs different from one's own' (Walker 2006: 11).

Howe (2009) refers to relationship-based social work as the skilled use of self. The ability to situate oneself with awareness and empathy so as to understand more fully the story, the issues and personal resources of those we work for and with, allow for strength, resilience and perceptiveness of the other to come through. How this applies between colleagues is critical to the negotiation process. In the fourth dialogue, the chair's explicit inclusion of the school nurse as the professional with 'key' information based on contact with the child cuts through a range of hierarchical perceptions and their subtle impact. As a result, feelings of insecurity or intimidation that the school nurse may feel are assuaged and crucial new information about Reece pulling his hair out is shared.

Howe (2008) highlights the relationship between the intrapersonal and the interpersonal that facilitates cognitive processes and manages the information while appreciating the significance of the exchanges. He helpfully defines emotionally intelligent individuals as those who are 'aware of and monitor their emotions; register and provide feedback on other people's emotions; use emotions to improve their reasoning; understand and analyse their own and other people's affective states; regulate and manage their own and other people's emotions and arousals; and co-operate and collaborate with others in mutually rewarding relationships' (2008: 14). The chair of the strategy meeting, in the fourth dialogue, comes close to achieving this. This level of emotional literacy, however, should be present in all attendees for the level of negotiation required. Munro refers to the 'group context' within which child protection decisions are made and highlights that 'groups are vulnerable to their own biases that lead to distorted reasoning. Their biggest failing is a desire to avoid conflict' (2008: 148). Being able to present a different perspective is crucial to the development of the broader sometimes richer and more textured story. Judging how and when to introduce these opinions requires careful consideration of place and context. Ability to operate comfortably and confidently in processes such as these is one of the hallmarks of emotional intelligence.

In his work on negotiation for health and social services professionals, Fletcher (1998) identifies nine key questions he believes are at the heart of the process which here are applied to the social worker at the meeting. They can provide an important framework for a negotiation strategy at any meeting and as such require a significant level of emotional intelligence:

1 **Who am I and what am I doing here?**
   I am Reece's social worker and I am here to represent him and report on the situation of risk to him.
2 **What do I want?**
   I want to establish if his family can address his weight problem so that his health is not compromised and his emotional well-being is restored.
3 **What am I prepared to give to get what I want?**
   I will provide a comprehensive report of my assessment.
4 **Who are they and what are they doing here?**
   They are my multi-agency colleagues who have important information to contribute to the process. I am concerned that they might see this as a children's services process, with less required of them.
5 **What do they want?**
   They also want Reece to be safe and well, but they may have additional concerns such as his educational achievement as well as preoccupations from their own work perspectives.
6 **What are they prepared to give to get what they want?**
   They will have reports to present which will reflect their professional and agency knowledge and responsibility, and their perspectives and opinions might be different from mine.
7 **How do I prepare the ground?**
   I will provide a clear report with an analysis of the risk and the protective factors.
8 **How do I manage the exchange?**
   I will invite discussion, listen and attend with care and challenge respect-fully. I won't shy away from debate.
9 **How do I assess the result?**
   The best result will be one that ensures as far as possible that the risk is addressed based on a thorough discussion of the available information and reflects the views and opinions around the table.

Social work is an arena where relationships should offer in large part a type of nurturance that holds and understands those feelings that are difficult and painful as well as those that are passionate and inspiring. Emotions are often the bedrock of the interaction, or as Howe states: 'They define the character of the professional relationship' (2008: 1). Morrison adds that 'emotions play a central role in decision making. The illusion that they can be somehow removed or put on ice while rational decision making is in progress is neither helpful nor possible' (2007: 256). Ability to negotiate from this perspective is more likely to bring people along because it presupposes a consideration of them and their views even if those views are different. It is also likely that account will be taken of their feelings and preoccupations, which can serve to take anger and hostility out of healthy disagreement. 'Emotionally intelligent people are good at negotiation and resolving conflicts. They are able to provide and receive emotional closeness, care and concern' (Howe 2008: 20).

Communication: methods

Respectful decision making

The aim of the strategy meeting in this script is to establish the nature and level of risk to Reece and ways to address it. How the information is shared, understood, assembled into facts and processed for the purpose of decision making must be conceptualized within a framework of legislation and procedure. As it is a meeting attended only by professionals, it offers opportunity for a particular type of discussion where an interrogation of the information and a sharing of expertise accommodates the expression of feelings, doubts and uncertainty as a source of information. It is a forum where participants can refer to their perception of what is happening as well as what they have observed and assessed. Ferguson (2011) pays particular attention to these 'intangibles' or 'uneasy feelings', providing as they can do, when appropriately explored, essential information for protecting children. Creating the right atmosphere through trust and openness, as well as accountability, provides for the distillation of this combination of knowledge. In this way a group of multi-agency professionals can engage in a meaningful way with the family and child in order to establish if abuse is taking place and if he or she is at risk of harm.

One useful method of communication that facilitates negotiation in a multi-agency child protection meeting draws largely on the principles of the exchange model of assessment combined with some procedural aspects as developed by Smale et al. (2000). Because the exchange model acknowledges the importance of shared expertise, partnership, participation and mutual understanding, it has clear applicability to a strategy meeting and to the type of communication required between professionals at the strategy meeting.

The model allows for the police officer to question whether the child's weight actually constitutes significant harm. As it is very often the case that families are not known to the police, as with Reece's family, the police officer attending will have the minimum of information such as a criminal records check and is in a good position to put questions to elicit new information or to offer a fresh perspective. The social worker can respond to questions about the family home and the impressions she formed on her visit, which may not be conclusive enough to form a judgement. Crucially the GP's attendance, in the fourth dialogue, allows for a factual report and informed opinion to be presented, enabling other professionals to question the implications of his diagnosis. Where the head teacher asserts that more support at an earlier stage from children's services might have helped to avoid this situation, the insinuation of blame can be acknowledged and the key point considered in the context of whether extra support now is sufficient to address the level of concern. Perhaps the school staff have additional information about the strengths of the family that are not available to the social worker given that she has only met the grandmother under difficult circumstances. An exchange of information such as this allows for negotiation and conciliation on the basis of shared expertise at all levels of professional experience. The school nurse's knowledge about Reece's expression of emotional distress is as important as the head teacher's assessment of Ms Murray when told about the quarrel in the playground.

This method also allows for the possibility of what White refers to as the 'argumentative flexibility to debate and make sense of what is being seen and recorded' (2009: 106). In her discussion about the dangers of information sharing and gathering in a climate of significant regulation directed towards workflows and gatekeeping, she makes a powerful case for valuing the processes that allow for interaction, interpretation and the type of communication that does not just get to the heart of the matter but ensures it is acted upon.

What can cause consternation to families, and unease for professionals, is when meetings about families are convened without their attendance. The idea that a lot of power is concentrated in such a meeting, and the possibility that professionals could run amok with their decision-making, is a not uncommon apprehension among parents and carers. It is very difficult to reassure families in circumstances such as these, particularly as they have to deal with their parenting being the subject of an investigation. However, the procedural nature of the process and anti-oppressive practice underpins accountability to the child, the family and the agencies. Procedural guidance and local protocols are there to protect against abuse of process. Assumptions must be challenged to avoid prejudice and discrimination creeping in. This is especially important when the *sense of things*, as referred to above, is being discussed. It is the role of the chair to ensure that appropriate checks and balances are maintained.

The approach–avoid axis

The approach–avoid axis is an additional communication method particularly relevant to analysis of group processes allowing, as it does, for reflection
on feelings and emotions. *Approach* behaviours include responding empa-
thetically to emotional information and reflection on one's own emotional
experience as a source of information. In contrast *avoid* behaviours rely on
'fleeing from emotional information, especially distress and anger, into
cognitive and factual realms and also include defensive practice such as
taking action to protect oneself or the organization rather than in the service
user's interests' (Koprowska 2007: 129).

In this case study, the social worker reflected on her emotional impressions and responses to the way Reece's grandmother, Rose Murray, interacted
with her, and responded to the concerns about Reece's obesity and absence
from school. Although the social worker had only met the grandmother once,
she formed an important judgement that the grandmother may be a proactive protector of Reece and as a member of the household must be included in
decision-making processes. The *approach* behaviour of the chair, in the fourth
dialogue, in acknowledging the busy schedules and time constraints of the
other professionals, facilitated an atmosphere of respect during the meeting:
'Approach behaviours are . . . about the atmosphere between people, not just
the number of minutes spent together. It stems from an aura of calm, not
haste; from interested attention, not preoccupation with the next task; from
eye contact rather than pen pushing. These are not inherently time consuming
but entail a level of personal containment and focus which are hard to achieve
when workers are stressed.' Because of the chair's approach, there was an
effective exchange of information between the participants at the meeting;
'approach behaviours generate more information than is strictly required,
uncover needs that cannot be met within current resources and may consume
more time' (Koprowska 2007: 129).

Communication: values and ethics

The centrality of the child's voice

The social worker did not get to speak to Reece directly, therefore she could
not represent his views at the strategy meeting. To ignore children's views is
to discriminate against them and therefore is an example of childism or
oppression of children. Article 12 of the UNCRC (United Nations 1989)
states that children have the right to have a say about decisions that affect
them and have their opinion heard. The Children Acts 1989 and 2004 also
enshrine the need for all agencies to listen to the views of the child and to

take them into account in decision-making, although professional judgement about what is in the child's best interests may override the child's own perceptions and wishes. Research by Cossar et al. (2011) of interviews with 19 children, who were the subject of child protection plans, demonstrated the specific importance of the social work relationship with the child: 'Young people who had a trusting relationship with the social worker felt that they were part of making positive changes happen in their families. By contrast, children and young people did not appreciate social workers whom they only saw at meetings and who they felt did not really know them.' Twelve of the children said they had seen the social worker on their own but these were more likely to be the older children: 'It is crucial that children who have a child protection plan are seen on their own by social workers, unless there is a specific reason not to do so, such as specialist communication needs. Seeing the child is a prerequisite for finding out the child's views' (Cossar et al. 2011: 63). The children said they valued being shown reports yet only 5 of the 19 children had been shown their child protection plan. Nelson's research of children's views emphasized that children need to be interviewed in neutral settings where they are free to respond. They want to be asked what their worries are about any investigation and to know how they can contribute to information presented at meetings (2007: 31–37). An Ofsted report (2011) also concluded, in a summary of findings from serious case reviews, that children's views were often excluded from the child protection process. This underlines the importance of working together with colleagues within statutory frameworks such as the strategy meeting.

Central to effective joint working is the proportionate sharing of information on a *need to know* basis across all services. The importance of the information and how it is interpreted and used is usually determined by the function and values of the service or agency. Deciding how and with whom information about children is shared is fraught with ethical and practice-based concerns, and more recently prompted significant controversy in the professional and public domain with the introduction of a national database for children. Economic constraints and charges of surveillance and intrusion, however, led to the abandonment of this initiative. Confidentiality is at the heart of what is understood to be both protective and problematic, not least how it is applied to children's information. Lishman (1993: 129) points out that 'issues of power, privacy and confidentiality have to be negotiated if the user of services is to benefit from the purpose of interdisciplinary interprofessional work, i.e. to receive an integrated service'. What must be made clear to practitioners and managers across all child protection agencies is the overriding responsibility to protect children and share information within child protection protocols. The sensitivity involved in sharing information should be reflected in the records so that clear accountability is maintained.

In the case of Reece, the fact that a number of professionals are aware of his vulnerability and potential risk is key to ensuring that concerns are shared and addressed. It is therefore critically important to examine what informs the communicative process of sharing information and agreeing on interpretation as well as formulating a plan of action arrived at through negotiation and professional consensus.

Not all adults or indeed parents behave in a protective way towards children. When risk of abuse is being investigated and a crime against a child is being considered, those potentially responsible for that crime cannot be part of that discussion, which is why Reece's mother is not permitted to attend the strategy meeting which is a professionals only forum. While the circumstances and the information may indicate that no crime has been committed, as identified by the police officer, it is only possible to establish this through the sharing of information and records in this forum. In social work with children, no professional meetings should take place without the knowledge or inclusion of parents and carers unless under the auspices of a Section 47 child protection investigation if to do so places the child at risk (Children Act 1989). Reece would be informed about the meeting as was appropriate for his age, understanding and best interests. If it was appropriate to inform him, he should have been spoken to on his own and asked how best his views might be shared at the meeting. He might suggest a specific trusted adult to represent his views and could provide a drawing, short letter or recording to be presented on his behalf. The child's perspective must be made available to the meeting and inform all decision-making.

Communication: the knowledge base

Childhood obesity

Reece's experience of living and coping in his 8-year-old world with the attendant problems of his weight is shared with a growing number of children classified as obese. The latest childhood obesity statistics, in the *Foresight Report*, identified that 'over 1 in 10 children aged between 2 and 10 are obese' (Aylott et al. 2008). This report predicted that 25 per cent of children would be obese by 2050 and the national clinical director for liver disease stated that 'thousands of children are at risk of fatal liver disease' (Donnelly 2011).

When health information with challenging messages enters the public domain, the debate tends to be situated and lines drawn around lifestyle issues, choice and accusations of interference by *the nanny state*. When children's health and well-being are involved, however, calls for a response become more far-reaching and influential. In 2007–2008, three cases of obese children in North Tyneside, Cumbria and Dundee were at the centre of media attention because of the children's services involvement with these families (Griffiths 2010). Most compelling, and perhaps more for reasons of voyeurism than child health and protection, images of a semi-naked 8-year-old boy, who weighed more than 14 stone, being assisted by his grandmother in basic personal tasks flashed across television screens on the national news on 26 February 2007. But however discomforting the viewing, such sensational programmes do have the effect of raising critical questions of risk and responsibility, not least the point at which childhood obesity becomes a child protection concern.

The question for the professionals at Reece's strategy meeting is whether his obesity constitutes a child protection risk. The chain of events that led to the referral from the head teacher originated with an incident in the school playground of a child being cruel to Reece on account of his weight. On further checking with other agencies it is established that Reece is actually known to the health agencies specifically due to his obesity. But an assiduous case analysis takes us further into the family circumstances and dynamics and what presents is that the management of Reece's obesity is directly connected to a parenting concern as a consequence of his mother's disengagement from the GP practice and her response to the incident. An additional and underlying vulnerability contributing to the assessment may be Ms Murray's learning disability, and the impact of this on her understanding of Reece's emotional fragility. Reece's grandmother appears to be supportive but she has not been able to influence Reece's return to school. Her capacity to stand up to her daughter is unknown.

Emerging therefore are a number of issues that, when combined, raise the threshold for risk identification. In complex child protection cases what often appears obvious masks the strength of view and perspective held by different participants in a statutory decision-making process. In the strategy meeting (third dialogue) the police officer, and to a degree the head teacher, are not convinced that the threshold has been met for ongoing child protection procedures to be implemented. But an examination of their rationale suggests their sympathy for Ms Murray's position in view of her learning disability and the demands of parenting. The police officer questions the appropriateness of the child protection process for a case of child obesity. The impact of the obesity on Reece's health and emotional well-being, and the likelihood of this continuing to go unaddressed, must be seen in the broadest context of the family with Reece firmly at the centre. Alexander et al. (2009: 136) support this and state that 'extreme childhood obesity may be viewed as a mirror image of severe non-organic failure to thrive. Parental neglect may be a causative factor in both circumstances. When suspicion of parental neglect arises, health care professionals may have both an ethical obligation and a statutory duty to notify child protection services.'

A group of British doctors agreed with a contextual position that obesity alone should not be considered a child protection issue and they advised social workers to intervene if parents fail to co-operate with treatment plans when their child's obesity presents a risk to health (Griffiths 2010). In the third dialogue, the fact that the GP does not attend places a difficult onus on the other participants to interpret his report problematizing further an already difficult negotiation.

The policy context: strategy meeting and working together

The detail of the purpose and process of the strategy discussion/meeting is outlined in *Working Together* statutory guidance (DfE 2010: 5.56/7/8) and is referred to in the script. It is essential that social workers are knowledgeable about this guidance to ensure children are protected. At the strategy meeting, detailed planning must include agreement between professionals about who should be interviewed, by whom, when and where, the need for a formal Achieving Best Evidence interview of the child (Ministry of Justice 2011), medical assessments/examinations, forensic retrieval and preservation of evidence and witness evidence. The needs of all children in the family or those in contact with an alleged perpetrator must be considered and account must be taken of the ethnicity of the child and family. The strategy meeting plans must be subject to review in order to ensure the continuity of the investigation.

The words *share and agree* feature prominently in the explanation and discussion of strategy meetings in *Working Together* (DfE 2010). Arriving at agreement in child protection meetings presupposes a discussion that includes a range of views, perspectives and positions with regard to the child, the family and the concerns. It is therefore a dynamic process often complicated by the strength of difference in professional opinion and entrenched positions assumed on the basis of role and profession, as well as loyalties and unrelated frustrations.

The agreement can be as dependent on the subtle but powerful interplay between professionals as on the information itself. It is, however, in this arena of divergent views, professional agendas and hierarchies that the necessary dissecting of facts and informed opinions ensures an agreed position for the safety of a child. It is to this process, in this context, that the communicative concept of negotiation is applied. It is difficult to imagine, except perhaps in the most straightforward of cases, that all of this could be accommodated in a phone call or strategy discussion as referred to above. When deciding what constitutes 'complex types of maltreatment' (DfE 2010: 154), or on the contrary straightforward investigations (Owen and Pritchard 1993), as the basis for having a strategy meeting rather than a phone discussion, it should be borne in mind that accountability, transparency, ownership and robustness are much more likely to be negotiated and assured in this crucial component of the child protection system when professionals sit down together and discuss, plan and allocate responsibility. Great care should be taken with the provision for flexibility and interpretation of procedure at the heart of a process addressing significant harm. Emphasis on timescales and performance indicators can become conflated with questions of seriousness and complexity and can lead to deeply unfavourable and unintended consequences.

Since the publication of the first among many *Working Together* policies (DHSS 1988), followed by the Children Acts 1989 and 2004 and a raft of additional related polices and procedures, the principle of co-operation and collaboration across and between agencies has been enshrined in social work practice. It has been clear that the outcome of any case depends significantly on the communication skills of professionals as much as their expertise: 'Safeguarding and promoting the welfare of children – and in particular protecting them from significant harm – depends on the effective joint working between agencies and professionals that have different roles' (DfE 2010). A child protection strategy meeting is the first formal opportunity in the child protection process for multi-agency professionals involved with the child to communicate about the risk of significant harm. In the context of cuts to services, this complex meeting may now be held solely by telephone discussion, thus denying professionals a setting where their negotiating skills can determine decisions and how they are made.

Multi-agency working

Much has been written about the work and practice of multi-agency teams both in social work generally and more specifically in relation to children's services (Morrison 2000; Glenny and Roaf 2008; Morris 2008). Multi-agency interprofessional teams are structured and constituted differently and over the past 15 years the changes, both structural and organizational, have left a bewildering array of terms and concepts. With reference to Reece's strategy meeting, the concentration will be on those teams whose members are drawn from different agencies and departments to co-operate and collaborate in addressing risk and making decisions. The effectiveness of their co-operation and ability to work together will depend on the organizational culture they come from, as well as their individual professional skill and commitment to a process of open discussion based on trust and respect.

In Foley and Rixon's work on changing children's services, they cite Frost's research in integrated teams and identify a list of some of the key themes that emerged (2008: 198–199; Frost 2005). Four are included here for their relevance to multi-agency work and underpinning the negotiation that needs to take place in complex child protection meetings: effective leadership; role clarity; a communication mindset; and inter-professional respect and trust. Without these as essential criteria on the front line, procedures are less likely to work and children will remain exposed to the vagaries of poor practice and highly compromised service delivery. The chair of Reece's strategy meeting must present a professional persona of leadership that communicates authority while at the same time presenting as respectful, open and eager to hear the contributions of multi-agency colleagues. The police officer must see himself as an active member of the team whose contribution extends beyond that of criminal investigator. Views and opinions he will offer from this perspective will carry the required weight and influence. Trust, established at the strategy meeting stage, will underpin potential joint working as the investigation or support work goes forward. This will also ensure consistency and commitment from this multi-agency team and is much more likely to convince and reassure the family. Ferguson (2011: 181) outlined a number of communication problems in multi-agency practice that have led to children not being protected such as when there is a different interpretation of risk as being higher or lower than the communicator intended.

Weaknesses in communication, no single agency having the complete picture, and professionals taking refuge in the communication of information rather than acting on it, are just some of the multi-agency problems drawn from serious case reviews by Reder et al. (1993). In December 2008, a 3-year-old child died of non-accidental injuries in Wolverhampton when in the care of adults, not the parents, who were known to other services. The executive summary stated: 'There is no evidence of effective communication or liaison between the different agencies involved with the mother or Child J at this time' and 'the original allegations of assault became "lost"' (WSCB 2011: 4.1.4, 4.2.4).

Recommendations regarding inter-agency communication from the two seminal public inquiries into the deaths of Victoria Climbié (Laming 2003) and Peter Connolly (HLSCB 2009) did not have the intended impact on those working with Child J, and the requirement and emphasis of the Children Act 2004 to co-operate through multi-agency arrangements based on effective communication, seemed in this context to have been awarded little relevance. The words 'time and time again' have a hollow tone. While the circumstances, contexts and even agencies are particular and distinct to individual cases, the overarching communication duties and requirements remain consistent.

Munro (2008: 149) analysed the process of group reasoning and identifies the tendency for consensus decision-making in child protection to 'reach agreement around a high or low risk assessment than a moderate one'. In the third dialogue which has a strong undercurrent of disagreement, in part driven by resentment and hostility, the strategy meeting decides that a child protection conference is necessary and plans for this to take place. In the fourth dialogue, however, there is more integrity in the multi-agency process: the meeting is well led and managed, trust and respect allow for information to be more thoroughly discussed and challenged, and this in turn allows for the strength of the family to be properly considered and potential for working with them to be evaluated. The decision could be classified as a moderate one in Munro's terms. Even though the case did not continue down a child protection path towards a conference there was acknowledgement that the family may not be able to respond to support and this was accounted for in the plan. 'Multi-agency work can be worthwhile if we allow the variety of different vocabularies, and a curiosity about them, alongside an understanding that we do not *find* facts we *make* them' (White 2009: 107).

Attendance of GPs at child protection meetings

In 2002 a report into the death of Lauren Wright concluded that a series of errors and a lack of best practice led to a failure to safeguard her (Brandon 2002). Lauren, aged six, died in May 2000 following the collapse of her digestive system as a result of a blow to the abdomen delivered by her mother. Lauren was examined by a GP, and subsequently by a paediatrician as part of the child protection enquiry. Numerous bruises of different ages were observed. The GP suspected child abuse, but the paediatrician's view was that bullying at school might have explained these. No multi-agency meeting took place to share, discuss and act on concerns for this child. The report strongly criticized the health service for their treatment of Lauren, specifically identifying failure to take ownership of child protection cases (Gillen 2002). More recently, the death of Peter Connolly in 2007 brought the issue back into the public domain and gave sharp focus yet again to the consequences for children when health professionals neglect to share professional ownership of child protection cases (CQC 2009). Tompsett et al. (2010), who conducted research about GPs and child protection responsibilities, found that some GPs were reluctant to refer to children's services as they lacked confidence in gaining a response and found it difficult to access social workers. When they did refer, they reported a lack of feedback about the case and they also had concerns about the impact of intervention on families. One finding of the study was a lack of reference to the views and wishes of children. GPs in the study also reported low attendance at child protection conferences, though provision of reports to conferences was higher than expected. Some suggested that conferences may be better informed by other health professionals who may hold more relevant information.

The Children Act 2004 places a duty on Local Safeguarding Children Boards to ensure local multi-agency arrangements are in place, and these arrangements must account for the attendance of GPs and relevant health professionals to take this responsibility seriously. Time constraints, competing priorities and venues for meetings are just some of the reasons cited for the lack of attendance. Flexibility in the practical arrangements might go some way towards addressing some of these problems. As the script above highlights, medical information is best interpreted by the appropriate health professional who would also be available to respond to queries and provide explanations as required. Given the complexity of the majority of child protection cases, and the health implications for all categories of abuse, the involvement of the GP is a clear priority. Munro (2008), in her discussion on group reasoning, referred to the propensity for group members to discount warnings if they came from people who are not present.

The fourth dialogue, with the GP attending, highlights too the importance of multi-agency discussion and the process of negotiation. This enriches exploration and allows for positions and views to be challenged in order to arrive at a shared understanding which in turn makes for safer, multi-agency owned and accountable decision-making that also has more chance of being implemented successfully.

CASE STUDY AND REFLECTION

Strategy meetings in the case of Victoria Climbié

'Strategy meetings were a key focus of scrutiny in the Victoria Climbié Inquiry' (Laming 2003). Victoria Climbié died in February 2000 aged 8 years following torture at the hands of her great aunt and her boyfriend who were both convicted for her murder. Laming conducted an inquiry into the case which reported in 2003.

Victoria was admitted to hospital by the London Borough of Brent Children's Services in June 1999 following the childminder's daughter taking her to hospital and disclosing that Victoria had bloodshot eyes and bruising on her arms, legs, buttocks and infected bruises on her fingers. Prior reported concerns from a distant relative about Victoria wetting herself constantly, not attending school and having cuts and bruises on her face did not inform the subsequent admission because checks were not made. The police used their powers of protection and Victoria stayed in hospital until the next day when she was discharged following a consultant's diagnosis that the injuries were accidental. Although neither Victoria, the carer, the childminder or her daughter were interviewed, the social worker redesignated the case as *child in need* rather than *child in need of protection*. There had been no Section 47 investigation and no strategy meeting. If such a meeting had taken place at the hospital, prior to discharge, the professionals would have been able to debate the circumstances of the case, analyse all available information and identify information as yet unknown such as the family history, which included Victoria's family in Africa and a period of time spent with the great aunt in France. The investigation would then have been planned to include protective legal safeguards, interviews of the child, family and referrer, a home visit, multi-agency communication, enquiries about her schooling and health care, and the medical information would have been situated within a social context. Crucially a decision would have been made about how safe it was to discharge Victoria when the explanations for her injuries remained unclear and had not been sought from the carer or the child. The inquiry concluded that 'no assessment of Victoria's needs was ever undertaken in response to the referral' (Laming 2003: 105).

Two strategy meetings were convened when the case was transferred to the London Borough of Haringey but both were ineffective in protecting Victoria. The inquiry concluded that deficiencies in the way the first strategy meeting was conducted were 'not an isolated example of poor practice' which 'would seem to be confirmed by the fact that many of the same faults are apparent in the second strategy meeting conducted a little over three months later' (Laming 2003: 199).

The first strategy meeting was in July 1999 after Victoria had been admitted to the North Middlesex hospital with severe burns to her head. The meeting was chaired by a senior practitioner rather than by a team manager, leading the inquiry to comment that 'the danger of inexperienced or inefficient chairmanship is well illustrated by Victoria's case' (Laming 2003: 199). There were 18 action points which were 'for the most part sound' (Laming 2003: 199). However, there was a lack of clarity about who was responsible for each decision and the minutes were not circulated which seriously affected implementation. There was no plan to convene a review strategy meeting in order to monitor the progress of the investigation. This lack of review caused the inquiry the greatest concern. Three different explanations for the burns as well as observation of old and new injuries were not explored with the carer and a seriously delayed arrival to hospital went unchallenged. Decisions about skeletal X-rays and photographs of injuries were never followed up and neither was there a paediatric overview relating to the prior hospital admission. There were decisions to make background checks, including with France and immigration authorities, and decisions to make checks on Victoria's schooling and her registration with a general practitioner. The inquiry stated that the strategy meeting should have taken place at the hospital in order to facilitate the attendance of the hospital staff. In fact, only four people attended the meeting, two from Haringey children's services, the police child abuse investigation officer and a social worker from the hospital. This lack of medical professional attendance led to much confusion about the status of the injuries and marks that were indicative of a dermatological condition such as scabies. Nurses had noted serious signs of neglect and emotional abuse in the relationship between Victoria and her great aunt and some injuries in the shape of a belt buckle, but these were not investigated by police and social workers and observations by those professionals close to the world of the child were not available to the meeting. There was no decision to proceed to a child protection conference and a social worker was allocated the case nine days after the hospital admission, when much of the initial concern had become diluted and lost from professional analysis.

The Haringey social worker was later barred from children's social work and one of the reasons was that she had failed to carry out the 15 decisions of the strategy meeting. She won her tribunal hearing, arguing, on this point, that the decisions should have been allocated to a range of professionals and they were not all her responsibility. No Section 47 joint investigation of harm was organized and no protection plan was in place. The social worker was inexperienced, untrained, poorly managed and following flawed protocols. She had a huge workload of 19 child protection cases and the case was defined by her manager as 'child in need' not 'child protection'. The social work approach was one of supporting a refugee family in accessing services rather than investigating allegations and evidence of serious child abuse.

The second strategy meeting made 15 decisions, in November 1999, following the aunt's referral of sexual abuse by her boyfriend. The inquiry referred to 'generally sensible action points' which if carried out would have 'gone a long way to establishing the danger that Victoria was in' (Laming 2003: 200). None of the action points were allocated to a specific individual and there were no stated timescales for completion and again no mechanism for review. There were just four people at the meeting, the chairperson, social worker and two police officers. Some of the previous decisions were repeated such as immigration checks and checks with France with no discussion of any progress made since the first decisions. There remained a lack of clarity about medical findings, although children's services were clear it was a family support case as medical records had confirmed the injuries were accidental (Laming 2003: 178). Three allegations of sexual abuse led to no Section 47 joint investigation and no formal interview of the child, carer or accused. It was concluded that the allegations were a ploy by the carer to obtain housing. Victoria herself, however, told the social worker, 'I'm not lying, I must tell you more. It is true.' The child went completely unheard partly because the social worker mistakenly thought, given that she was untrained in investigative interviewing, that she should not speak with Victoria. She could, of course, have asked a few open questions to clarify what Victoria was saying. This approach would not have contaminated a subsequent Achieving Best Evidence formal recorded interview (Ministry of Justice 2011).

If there had been a strategy meeting at the time of the first hospital admission which had steered a Section 47 investigation and led to a child protection conference then the following would have taken place:

- When the family moved to Haringey there would have been a transfer conference. This would have led to continuity of information sharing and protective planning.
- A series of review strategy meetings as further information came to light would have enabled new facts to be analysed in the context of old physical injuries as well as observations of neglect and emotional harm.
- Professionals in each agency would have been identified as having clear focused responsibilities.
- A named paediatrician would have collated all medical information, X-ray findings and photographic evidence and provided the social worker and police with a coherent summary of findings to guide the investigation.
- An education social worker would have explored the reasons for Victoria not being allocated to a school.
- Nurses and ward staff would have had a clear channel for reporting their concerns to a co-ordinated investigative team.
- The police and social worker would have examined the evidence checking forensically to see if injuries and explanations matched or not. They would also have searched for implements in the home which might have matched and explained the range of unusual and serious marks on Victoria's body.
- The outcome of interviews with the referrers, childminder, relative and with the great aunt and her boyfriend as well as a formal interview of Victoria using an interpreter, as English was her third language, would have informed the analysis of known facts.
- Decisions about discharge from hospital, return home and the child's safety would have been multi-agency decisions.

In the inquiry, Laming (2003:205) suggested that social workers practice 'respectful uncertainty' being confident to challenge and critically evaluate information they receive.

Laming said he was 'amazed that nobody in any of the key agencies had the presence of mind to follow what are relatively straightforward procedures on how to respond to a child about whom there is concern of deliberate harm' (Laming 2003: 4). It is these procedures that provide the structures within which effective challenge and negotiation can take place. There was evidence available throughout this case which if properly co-ordinated and analysed by professionals working together in compliance with statutory procedures could have led to protective action.

Questions to aid reflection

Drawing on the knowledge presented in this chapter and your learning from analysis of the script consider the following questions:

 What is the importance of face-to-face contact between professionals from different agencies in the negotiation process?

 How is respectful uncertainty *used to enhance professional communication in the strategy meeting?*

 How is the child's view best represented in formal child protection processes?

 What specific knowledge base best informs a social worker's communication with a parent with a learning disability?

 Identify the essential components of a strategy meeting that underpin sound, statutory multi-agency decision-making?

Agencies and websites

Social workers need to be informed about the key agencies involved in this area of work so that they know where to access specialist advice and support.

Ann Craft Trust Centre for Social Work. National association for the protection from abuse of children and adults with learning disabilities. www.anncrafttrust.org

Childhood Obesity National Support Team (CONST). http://www.dh.gov.uk/en/Publichealth/Obesity/index.htm

Respond. Challenges vulnerability and sexual abuse in the lives of people with learning disabilities. www.respond.org.uk

Recommended reading

Cleaver, H. and Nicholson, D. (2007) *Parental Learning Disability and Children's Needs: Family Experiences and Effective Practice*. London: Jessica Kingsley Publishers.

Department for Education (2010) *Working Together to Safeguard Children: A Guide to Inter-agency Working to Safeguard and Promote the Welfare of Children.* London: The Stationery Office.

Glenny, G. and Roaf, C. (2008) *Multiprofessional Communication: Making Systems Work for Children.* Maidenhead: Open University Press.

Howe, D. (2008) *The Emotionally Intelligent Social Worker.* Basingstoke: Palgrave Macmillan.

McGaw, S. and Newman, T. (2005) *What Works for Parents with Learning Disabilities?* Available from: http://www.barnardos.org.uk/what_works_for_ parents_with_learning_disabiliities_publications_tracked.pdf

Morrison, T. (2007) Emotional intelligence, emotion and social work: context, characteristics, complications and contribution, *British Journal of Social Work,* 37(2): 245–263.

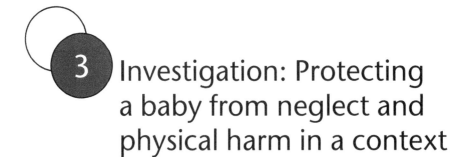

3 Investigation: Protecting a baby from neglect and physical harm in a context of parental resistance

Introduction

Chapter content

Since the mid-1990s the skills of investigation and assessment have become confused in policy and practice guidance. There has been a shift away from policy focused on protecting children which has resulted in a change of professional language (Munro and Calder 2005). Wattam commented that, 'those who have the power to define the terms have the power to shape the discourse' (1996: 192). Policy generally now refers to *assessment, need, concern* and *safeguarding* instead of *investigation, risk, abuse* and *protection*. Parton commented that the concept of *safeguarding* is that of minimization of harm and promotion of well-being rather than protection from significant harm (2006: 7).

This chapter stresses the importance of focusing communication and action on the need to protect the child from harm. Studies have shown that individual social workers do understand the importance of language and dialogue but are less 'conscious of the impact of the processes which created their, *special* professional language on either themselves or on the service users on whom they impose the discourse' (Gregory and Holloway 2005: 50). In this script and case study, the social workers did not understand the political changes which underpinned and steered their work away from their prime duty to protect the child. Instead, support of the parent took precedence. There was, therefore, an emphasis on parental strengths at the expense of the child's vulnerability. Vojak commented that 'social service practitioners and theorists studying the use of language in the helping professions have noted how institutionalized jargon reflects prevailing ideological, political and economic interests, and thus maintains existing power relations' (2009: 937).

In this chapter, the distinction is made between investigation and assessment and the focus is the investigation of child abuse conducted by social workers with police and other agencies through *Working Together* statutory guidance (DfE 2010). The script demonstrates the dynamics sometimes used by parents and carers to divert professional attention from the abuse of children. Numerous child abuse inquiries have shown that social workers often collude with these dynamics through processes of professional dangerousness. Theories and methods of communication that help to inform efforts to counter these avoidant responses are outlined with reference to the script. The chapter concludes with the case study of Peter Connolly on which the script was based although it differs in much of the detail.

Summary of the script

The first and second dialogues present the social worker, Patti, on a home visit to a parent, Abi, who seemingly co-operates, but in fact places many obstacles in the way of effective communication, diverts Patti's attention and thereby blocks her professional focus on the needs of Darren, the child. In the third dialogue (A) Patti, on a second home visit, continues to be ineffective in her communication to protect Darren. In the alternative dialogue (third dialogue B) Patti demonstrates her communication skills in keeping the focus on Darren and his need for safety. This approach, respectful of the parent but retaining the centrality of the child's needs, enables and informs the progression of the multi-agency child protection investigation.

The script: Patti, the social worker, communicates with Abi, mother of 16-month-old Darren during the process of an investigation of alleged child abuse

Setting the scene

The case involved 28-year-old Abi Morrissey and her then 16-month-old son Darren who had been cause for concern almost since he was born. When six weeks old he attended clinic with a nappy rash and later again presented with diarrhoea and vomiting. Similar incidents reoccurred and the health visitor became concerned. Abi took Darren, age seven months, to the doctor who noted marks and bruises on Darren's head and chest. Abi said he had fallen down the stairs. When he was nine months old, Darren attended hospital with bluish colouring over the bridge of his nose and serious bruising to the cheek and forehead. Police arrested Abi who gave a number of inconsistent reasons not matching the injuries. She said the causes were by the family dog, Darren falling onto his toys and also banging his head on the fireplace. Abi said Darren had a tendency to bang his head against the bars of his cot. There was no evidence of *easy bruising syndrome* which provides a medical explanation for bruises in children who have the condition.

Darren was placed with foster carers for a period and his name was subject to a child protection plan under the categories of neglect and physical abuse – although medical investigations, to suggest Darren was actually hit by an adult, were inconclusive. The professionals did think there were possibilities for improvement in Abi's parenting. Abi's attitude towards Darren started to improve, a community psychiatric nurse visited regularly for Abi's sporadic depression and she agreed to attend a Family Centre with Darren twice a week. She was also attending parenting classes once a week and a care worker from her local church visited weekly.

Both the Family Centre worker and the health visitor noted that Darren often presented with poor hygiene and was dressed inappropriately for the weather. Although some improvements were noted in relation to a reduction of concerning incidents, attendance at the Family Centre was sporadic with Abi often attending alone. Staff were also concerned that Darren was underweight for his age, but ate ravenously when he came to the Family Centre.

Abi lived on her own in a council property. The parenting class manager had noticed that Abi now had a new boyfriend since her husband had left who sometimes brought Darren to the centre.

First dialogue

Patti visits Abi at home. The house smells of urine. Old magazines and half-empty jars of baby food are strewn around. The carpet was sticky and stained, and on the couch were half-wet disposable nappies and a large rottweiler dog. Patti did not know how dangerous the dog might be and felt frightened.

Abi: [*Smiles*] Come in. You must be Patti.

Patti: Hello.

Abi: Oh look, thanks for coming. I know how busy you must be and I do appreciate you coming today.

Patti: Well the main reason I have come, as I'm sure you're aware is . . .

Abi: Yeah well, come in first, eh. Sorry the place is a bit of a tip. You do think it's a tip don't you? Oh whatever must you think of me? I feel awful. I was going to tidy up. I thought the new social worker is coming this afternoon. I have to tidy up. But well, see . . .

Patti: I'd be concerned that your dog is nuzzling those jars of baby food. I'd be concerned for the baby's health and . . .

Abi: It isn't the baby that's eating them is it, though? It's this fella here isn't it? [*Pats dog*] Isn't it Tiger? Darren doesn't eat baby food. I cook him proper stuff like they say at the Family Centre.

Patti: The point I'm making is . . .

Abi: You're right. I apologize. You're right. I need to try harder. I was gonna tidy up. Hygiene. The place is a tip, no place to bring up a baby. Only – well! Not been feeling well lately.

Patti: Oh I'm sorry to . . .

Comment

Abi is continually distracting Patti from her core role in protecting Darren. She begins by being friendly and welcoming thus creating an illusion of co-operation. She then acknowledges the state of the house and pre-empts Patti's comments by interjecting with her own seeming acceptance of the problem. This aspect of professional dangerousness is *false compliance*. A parent or carer presents as being in agreement with the social worker and diverts professional attention away from harm to the child. Abi already has Patti apologizing to her as if it is Patti who is causing the problem. Patti needs to gain control of the interview from the start and keep Darren's safety central. This could be achieved by confronting the immediacy of the visit and making reflective comments on what was happening in the 'here and now', e.g. 'Abi you keep interrupting me and it's really important that you listen to what I am saying . . .' or 'Yes Abi you are right the place is a terrible mess and Darren is at risk from the dog and from all the dirt. You are right this is no place to bring up a baby – you have said it yourself so what are you going to do about it?'

Abi: After Darren was born I got depressed. I'm under Dr Gerard for it. You know him?

Patti: I'm afraid I've never . . .

Abi: He's a senior consultant psychiatrist. Lovely man. Abi, he says, you've got to think about yourself. He blames my husband who used to knock me about. I mean that's what started it all. It's not the physical stuff is it? It's all the emotion. You love a man and you give him everything, you have his children and how does he repay you? He beats you up. That's what started it all. Been depressed for months. Dr Gerard says I've had an unhappy childhood because my mother was an alcoholic and my Dad left us. I get depressed real bad sometimes.

Patti: Oh I'm sorry to hear that.

Comment

Patti is now showing empathy with Abi but the care of Darren has not been addressed and is secondary to Abi's own problems. She could acknowledge Abi's difficulties and then swiftly move on to the reason for the visit, e.g. 'I'm sorry you are having such a hard time Abi but we really must talk about Darren now.' Patti could also acknowledge the statements about depression to draw attention to the neglectful and harmful parenting, e.g. 'Abi I know you feel depressed. How do you think that is affecting your care of Darren? It's really important I understand how you are feeling because then I will be able to better understand what Darren is going through.'

Abi: [*Looks her up and down aggressively*] Yeah. Still he's gone now. [*Shouts*] Tiger come and meet the new social worker. Here boy come on. [*to Patti*] Don't worry he won't bite. He's as gentle as a lamb really. Down Tiger. Don't jump all over Patti whatever will she think . . .

Patti: I'd rather you put him out if that's alright?

Abi: Oh yeah, sure. He normally stays outside but what with it raining and everything. He hates the rain.

Patti: It's just that I'd rather conduct this interview . . .

Patti: Oh yes, you're right. Sorry. Out Tiger. [*Kicks dog*] You are scaring the poor social worker. There. Safe now eh?

Patti: Thank you.

Comment

Patti rightly challenged the presence of the dog which she knew was affecting her ability to conduct the interview effectively. She should have been more assertive, e.g. 'Please Abi, put the dog outside so that we can talk about Darren. I cannot continue this interview with the dog jumping all over me and we need to talk about Darren.'

Abi: Yeah, sorry about that. Your first visit and I'm in a holy mess. Sorry. Don't know what you must think. I promised myself that I would show you how good a mother I can be and look the house is a complete tip and the dog is running riot everywhere.

Patti: Right well . . .

Abi: Because I do try hard. I do want to work with you like they said at that meeting. I'd do anything to have Darren's name taken off that list. Anything . . .!

Patti: Yes.

Abi: [*Cries*] They said I hit him. I never hit him. I wouldn't do a thing like that. [*Covers face*] I never hit him. Honestly . . . He hit himself on the fireplace. I'm sure he did. [*Snivels*] That's what Marcia said. It was an accident. Marcia bought me a fireguard. Marcia is from the church. She's a care worker and she's been ever so good. Don't know what I'd have done without her and my friends from the church.

Patti: Perhaps we should sit down and have a chat there are one or two things . . .

Comment

Patti misses a cue here. Abi provides a rationale for the injuries which a child protection doctor has already ruled out because the explanations were inconsistent with the visible marks. Patti should have reiterated that the doctors had not accepted the fireplace explanation, that the cause of the injuries was not known and therefore still of concern, e.g. 'Abi, you are saying that you did not hit Darren but we do not understand what caused his injuries. He could not have done them himself and your explanations do not fit the injuries. I know you care about Darren, so tell me – if you didn't cause these marks who else do you think might have harmed him?'

Abi: Only it was a difficult time then you know. Can't remember a lot about all that. I was on a lot of tablets then, for depression. I think they frazzle your mind. Anyway I can't remember. Complete blank.

Patti: Right.

Abi: But you needn't worry I wouldn't do that ever. Hit him I mean. Not ever. I mean I lie awake nights thinking about what they said I might have done to that poor lad. He's all I got. I'm lucky to have him. I promise, I really am going to make this better – work really hard.

Patti: Yes. Abi we need to talk about few things. One of the things you agreed to do . . .

Abi: Yeah?

Patti: Well we did say, didn't we, that we'd like you to take Darren to see the health visitor?

Abi: I did, didn't I? This morning.

Patti: Really?

Abi: Yeah, well no. What am I saying'? No, I went to the health centre but there was a queue a mile long and I don't like him waiting around at that health centre. He gets crotchety and I'm always worried he might catch something. Either it's a runny nose or a pain in his tummy. And he's a little devil for bruises. Always banging into things. And he bruises so easy. That's what the doctor said. I expect you read that in the report.

Patti: [*Confused*] OK Abi. It's really important that you take Darren to see the health visitor regularly . . .

Abi: How about first thing tomorrow when it's less crowded first thing? We don't have to wait around so long then.

Patti: Well that would be really useful if you could take Darren along tomorrow . . .

Abi: I will for sure, first thing.

Patti: Because then the health visitor can . . .

Comment

Patti has tried to state the importance of the health checks. She should make clear to Abi that it is her professional role to speak to the health visitor and make sure Abi took Darren to the appointment. She needs to emphasize that this is part of the child protection plan. It isn't enough to say, 'that would be really useful' she should say, e.g. 'Abi, as part of the protection plan you are required to take Darren to see the health visitor and you will find her advice helpful.' A child protection doctor had already ruled out the *easy bruising syndrome*. Therefore Patti should have challenged Abi's assertion that Darren bruised easily.

Abi: I do understand that. Very first thing. But I need a little help. I wonder whether you could –

Patti: Yes?

Abi: [*Jolly*] Darren is such a little devil, well I mean he's so playful. He thinks everything is a big laugh but when he goes to that supermarket he causes disaster. Last time he pulled all the cola on the floor. What I'm saying is that I have a real problem taking Darren shopping because I can't control him. And there have been occasions, not recently, when I've left him asleep in his cot while I get a quick taxi to the supermarket.

Patti: You left him alone in his cot?

Abi: No. No! I wouldn't leave him on his own. Declan's here. He's my friend who comes round sometimes doing his handyman stuff. But he doesn't really like to look after Darren unless he's asleep or quiet. Not the most patient guy in the world. I haven't done it in the longest time though. So it's not a problem now. Well it would be if I still went to the supermarket which I don't. Though I'd like to. It's cheaper. Would you like some tea?

Patti: No thanks. Is Declan a boyfriend?

Abi: Declan. Oh no! [*Mimicking Patti*] Is Declan a boyfriend? No I don't have a partner as it goes.

Patti: I was just trying to establish . . .

Abi: Oh yeah I know you've got to ask questions. That's your job isn't it?

Patti: Does he live here?

Abi: Live here? No he doesn't live here. He has his own flat in North Road.

Patti: Abi . . . I just wanted . . .

Abi: See Declan's just a friend. I see him at church. We go there a lot together. He helped me move in. You know fixing things.

Patti: I do need to know a full family picture.

Abi: Right 'course you do. But my problem is I need to shop online and I need a fiver for the delivery. Can social services help with that?

Patti: Well. I'd need to make some . . .

Abi: Only it would be a big help. Because you people have been wonderful helping me and Darren. When I went to the conference and you all said he could come back home I could've cried I was that happy. [*Cries*] I'm sorry. I just get a bit upset when I think . . . breaks my heart sometimes . . . sorry.

Patti: Well I'll certainly make some enquiries. And . . . Right. Look Abi. There are a couple of things we need to talk about.

Abi: I suppose you'll be wanting to inspect things – kitchen, bedroom, stuff like that.

Patti: Sorry? Why would I . . .?

Abi: Well isn't that what you're supposed to do? Make sure the baby's cot is clean and the kitchen's hygienic. All that. And I'm not really ready. The place is really a mess isn't it? Whatever will you think of me?

Patti: Abi I don't want to inspect the beds.

Abi: Only I don't want you to think I'm hiding anything, 'cos you know I have to prove myself haven't I? Prove I can be a good mother to Darren.

Patti: I really wanted to take a look at Darren.

Abi: Darren?

Patti: Yes.

Abi: Oh no!

Patti: What?

Abi: Only well. Well Darren's out. Sorry.

Patti: Darren's out! Where?

Abi: Mark and Gillian have taken him to the park. He loves that park and the swings. [*Laughs*] I'd put a swing in here if I could.

Patti: Yes. So. . . . Who are?

Patti/Abi: Mark and Gillian?

Abi: They're my friends from the church.

Patti: What time will they . . .?

Abi: I do chunter on, don't I? I suppose I get nervous with authority. I really want to show everyone that I can be a good mother to Darren. I really want to try hard. I suppose that's why I react the way I do. I suppose I'm really nervous underneath. Did you say 'yes' to the tea?

Patti: What time will . . .?

Comment

Abi has managed to get Patti on the defensive. She has flitted from one topic to another, constantly interrupting and inviting her to have tea. Patti needs to take control of the interview and impose a structure. The first aspect to address is whether or not Abi is leaving Darren on his own in the cot as she has said. Instead of avoiding the subject, Patti needs to make it possible for Abi to explore further her neglect of Darren, e.g. 'Abi you just said you were leaving Darren alone in his cot. You must be quite stressed out to be doing that. Is shopping really that bad? Tell me more about what happens.' In relation to Declan, Patti does need to know about adults in the household and potentially very dangerous routines. She could employ a line of questioning that does not immediately offend Abi, thereby terminating the visit. She could thank Abi for his address and explain that she will need to ask her police colleague to check it out and that this is routine when a child is the subject of a protection plan. When Abi suggests Patti might like to look at the rooms in the house Patti responds defensively. This is a classic dynamic in *false compliance* when the parent/carer gets in first to call the bluff of the social worker. Patti should have responded, 'Yes Abi you are absolutely right I do need to look around the bedrooms and kitchen. You probably remember that was a decision at the conference that my visits include checking rooms. Again, I know it is intrusive but that's quite usual where there are worries about neglect of a child.' Patti cautiously says she wants to take a look at Darren. Again, she needed to be more assertive, e.g. 'Abi where is Darren? I haven't seen him or heard him since I arrived. I need to see him.'

Abi: How old are you, Patti?
Patti: I'm 23 but actually . . .
Abi: And did you say you were married?
Patti: Er no.
Abi: Any children?
Patti: Er . . . no. Do you like going to the Family Centre, Abi? Sally says you never seem to want to get too involved when you go there.
Abi: Oh I do. I really like going to that Family Centre. They're ever so good. They teach me . . .
Patti: Sally says she had to have a word with you a couple of weeks ago about you seeming to prefer playing with your mobile phone rather than getting involved with activities.
Abi: Yeah, sorry. It's just that, well, I get nervous really, all those mums. I feel a bit intimidated. But I do like going. I've learnt a lot about parenting.
Patti: You have missed a lot of days. Your attendance there is not . . .
Abi: You know what that is. That's routine. I mean with moving and everything. And you know being nervous. Once I get into a routine I'll be fine.
Patti: The Family Centre is important Abi . . .
Abi: Oh Patti, I know, I know. And you're right I really have to try harder. I want my baby's name off that list don't I? Whatever must you think? All these tears.

The dog comes into the room and jumps up at Patti.

Abi: Down Tiger, down. Don't worry, he's only growling at you because you're new. He won't bite you or anything. [*Shouts*] Jago! Jago! Come and get this hound. The social worker is scared. Get upstairs to Jago. [*Shouts*] Let him in your room, Jago.

As Abi opened the door to force the dog out Patti glimpsed a tall man dressed in a combat suit. He had a large jagged knife fastened to his belt. He looked at her guiltily as though he was surprised to see Patti.

Patti: Abi . . . Jago . . . is *he* a boyfriend?

Abi: What, Jago? [*Laughs*] No Jago is just a friend. No he is not a boyfriend or anything. He's just a friend.

Patti: From the church?

Abi: Well, no he's not really from the church. Well sort of . . . he's just a friend.

Patti: He was upstairs.

Abi: No . . . Well yeah well he was fixing something for me 'cos housing take weeks to come round. Declan don't know much about electrics but Jago is very good at that sort of thing. He used to do it for a living.

Patti: Right. But you said your room.

Abi: What?

Patti: You said, 'Let him in your room.'

Abi: Yeah, well I meant the room he was working in.

Patti: But he seems to know er . . . Tiger.

Abi: Yeah, he takes Tiger out all the time. He likes dogs. Bit of a military man is Jago. And I think he'd love a dog of his own. Look Patti, he doesn't live here.

Patti: Abi look . . .

Abi: I live here on my own with Darren. Honest. [*Pause*] You can come round and check anytime. You must be really confused with all these men around. Must look really awful.

Patti: Look Abi, all I want to do is establish a clear picture of who is in the home.

Abi: Yeah sorry. When you rang I thought you just wanted a chat with me, sort things out and that. Only if you wanted to see Darren you should have said – it wouldn't have been a problem. You just said you wanted to see me. A bit of a mix up really. Next time you come I'll make really sure Darren is here. Shall we make another appointment?

Patti: How about this afternoon?

Abi: Yeah that would be great.

Patti: Good, how about . . .?

Abi: Oh no!

Patti: What?

Abi: Could you come after teatime 'cos I've got to go out? Well, it's my Dad. He's not well. Thing is he's dying and I do feel I should be there as often as I can.

Patti: Oh Abi, I'm sorry to hear that.

Comment

Abi has now confused Patti, leading her to believe that she had not made the purpose of the visit clear even though the details of the plan were outlined at the conference. Abi hardly allows Patti to complete a sentence, shifts the conversation to Patti's own life circumstances and to Abi's father's alleged illness. When asked about her children, Patti could have steered the conversation back to the points needing to be explored, e.g. 'I'm here to talk about you and Darren today, not about me, and now I want to know why you have missed so many appointments at the centre. You are required to take Darren there regularly and they do let me know what's going on. If it's difficult for you then we need to think about how to get you there.'

Second dialogue

> *Patti returns to the house that afternoon and arrives just as Abi is on her way out with Darren in the buggy.*

Abi: So you think Darren's fine then? Nothing bad to report? Will you write a report? Will I be able to see it?

Patti: Well naturally . . . Abi there are some things we need to talk about.

Abi: Sure, yeah no problem. But not today though. I have an appointment with my CPN.

Patti: Right.

Abi: But look, why don't you come down to the Family Centre on Thursday. We can have a long chat. How about that?

Patti: [*Encouraged*] Yes that would be . . .

Abi: I took him round to the clinic last week. Health visitor said he was fine. Little bit underweight – but coming along nicely. That's what the health visitor said. Coming along just fine.

Alternative dialogues

In the next section two alternative dialogues are explored. The first continues in the same mode of communication as presented in dialogues 1 and 2. The second offers an example of an investigative approach. As you read these two different methods of communication give consideration to Patti's perspective on:

- the sense of fear and discomfort in the family home
- the social worker's responsibility to see Darren despite the distractions presented by Abi
- a difficulty in retaining a focus on the child at risk of harm
- an uncertainty about her statutory protective role and methods of Section 47 joint investigation
- her helplessness in the face of the men and dog in the household
- the need to ensure she obtains quality supervision and training.

Third dialogue (A)

Patti visits Abi again after a period when Abi has been uncontactable. Patti has become increasingly frantic, making phone calls and calling at the house even in the evenings but getting no response.

Abi: Come in. Good to see you. Tea? I'll put the kettle on. Darren's fast asleep in his buggy. I'll take him down to the Family Centre when he's awake.

Patti: Abi, where've you been? I've been really worried.

Abi: I've been to see my uncle. He's really ill. He's dying.

Patti: Why didn't you say you were going away?

Abi: I did. Oh come on, we all look after our family, yeah. It's blood. I mean I'm entitled to go and look after a sick uncle. You're not going to deny me that?

Patti: No, it's just that . . . you could've phoned.

Abi: I would've done only I thought you would be busy enough without me phoning you up all the time. You'll want to see Darren then. He's still in his buggy I'm afraid.

Abi pulls Patti over to where Darren lies in his buggy asleep. He looks thin and pale and is sleeping restlessly.

Abi: [*Whispers*] I would be very grateful if you wouldn't wake him. He's very tired. That gauze on his fingers is where he trapped them in the caravan door. Poor little mite.

Patti: Abi what's that? What's that on his scalp?

Abi: [*Whispers*] Shusssh. [*Smiles*] It's only chocolate. He licks at it when he gets bored and rubs it in his head.

Patti: No, not that. The cream. It's gone all flaky.

Abi: The doctor gave it me because he had sores. Yeah, I think he may have caught lice. Only a precaution. Have to keep it on for 24 hours. I'll have to get a move on. I've got an appointment with the CPN.

Third dialogue (B)

Abi: Come in. Good to see you. Tea? I'll put the kettle on. Darren's fast asleep in his buggy. I'll take him down to the Family Centre when he's awake.

Patti: Yes, please do put the kettle on, I'd love a cup of tea. We've got a bit of time before the Family Centre opens.

Abi makes tea and gives a cup to Patti.

Patti: Thanks Abi. Did you realize I have been trying to contact you for over a week? Darren is the subject of a child protection plan which means I have to know where he is staying.

Abi: I've been to see my uncle. He's really ill. He's dying.

Patti: I'm sorry to hear that Abi but my main consideration is for Darren's safety. If you had let me know your address there would have been no problem, but I had no idea where you and Darren were – you must realize that caused a great deal of concern for him?

Abi: Oh come on, we all look after our family, yeah. It's blood. I mean I'm entitled to go and look after a sick uncle. You're not going to deny me that?

Patti: It's really important that you see your family, but it is my responsibility to monitor the care of Darren which I have to do because he is on a child protection plan. That's serious Abi, because he has had numbers of unusual, unexplained injuries and you had not been caring for him properly.

Abi: I would've done only I thought you were busy enough without me phoning you up all the time. You'll want to see Darren then? He's still in his buggy I'm afraid.

Abi pulls Patti over to where Darren lies in his buggy asleep. He looks thin and pale and is sleeping restlessly.

Abi: [*Whispers*] I would be very grateful if you wouldn't wake him. He's very tired. That gauze on his fingers is where he trapped them in the caravan door. Poor little mite.

Patti: I can't take any risks now with Darren. Any new marks, sores or injuries must be examined by the child protection doctor, Dr Matthews, who saw him in hospital on the first occasion he had injuries. I will organize an appointment today. I realize he may have had an accident with his finger and that you covered it with a bandage, but I need to make sure that it was an accident as you say. Being the subject of a child protection plan means that your care of Darren is being monitored to make sure he is OK. I know you want the best for Darren, so it really is in both his and your interest to get him checked out by a specialist doctor. Abi, he really is covered in chocolate isn't he? I can hardly see his face through it. Please wipe it clean now so that I can see him properly.

Abi: [*Whispers*] Shusssh [*Smiles*] It's only chocolate. He licks at it when he gets bored and rubs it in his head.

Patti: The cream seems to have gone all flaky. Must be very irritating for him.

Abi: The doctor gave me cream because he had sores. Yeah, I think he may have caught lice. Only a precaution. Have to keep it on for 24 hours. I'll have to get a move on. I have got an appointment with the CPN.

Patti: I'm sorry Abi, but I'm not happy with all this. I have decided that we must now take Darren to the hospital clinic straight away to have him checked out by Dr Matthews. I will call your CPN and explain that you cannot see her today. I'm sure she will rearrange the appointment soon. You see Abi, your needs are important but Darren has to come first and it's my job to make sure of that.

Abi: You really make a fuss don't you? There's nothing wrong with him, but OK then we'd better get on and get it over with so I can get back and make the tea 'cos Declan's going to be back from work as hungry as anything.

Patti: I'm going to have to ask the police to make some checks on Declan because he visits the home often. That's what happens when a child protection plan is in place. The conference decision was for checks to be made on all adults who have contact with Darren.

Abi: Declan will be right pissed off about that. You don't even know his full name or anything. Oh well, do what you like, you will anyway, there's no stopping you. Just it makes things a hundred times worse for me and Darren.

Patti: If you are worried Abi, we need to think about keeping you and Darren safe. I can speak with the police about that if you want me to and I can find you a refuge, but you need to learn to trust me and let me help you if that's the case. Now let's get in my car and get to the clinic before it closes.

Comment

In this dialogue Patti demonstrates her ability to communicate in order to progress the child protection investigation. She speaks to Abi sensitively and clearly always bringing the subject back to the protection of Darren without communicating in a punitive and stigmatizing way. This approach provides an opportunity for Abi to stop being defensive, and to express fear about Declan. Patti was then able to provide Abi with options for her and Darren to find safety together. This is the first time that Abi allows herself to trust Patti sufficiently and begin to acknowledge her difficulties. This is just a beginning but the door has opened for Abi and Darren together to find safety with social work involvement.

Communication: theory

Transmission theory

Communication is a process of transmitting a message from one person to another, and in this case study between Patti and Abi. A range of factors can block the effectiveness of this transmission. Here, the *noise* or *interference* preventing Patti's message being received by Abi was primarily Abi's resistance to compliance with the protection plan and ensuring the safety of her child. This was evident in her constant interruptions, distractions, false compliance and avoidance tactics. She also, after hearing the message from Patti, continued to resist, often repeating or pre-empting Patti's communications leading to further miscommunication (Shannon and Weaver 1964). Communication, however, is more than a message from one person to another because, 'it is never enough for the speaker to send the message, the recipient has to receive it and understand it as intended' (Calder 2008: 71; Reder and Duncan 2003). Effective communication is the responsibility of both the message initiator and the receiver. 'It is a mind-set, a skill that can be learned, rehearsed and refined' (Calder 2008: 72). Errors take place when the message is misunderstood and this is a key finding in many child abuse inquiries (Munro 1999).

Perceptual screens

Interference may also be in the form of ideologies and what are referred to as *perceptual screens* which may affect the capacity or willingness of the recipient to understand the message as intended (Lasswell 1948). Allen and Langford refer to this as selective perception which 'allows us to look for sense and patterns in our social interactions as well as choosing to focus on certain phenomena' (2008: 23).

Patti defined her role as one of *family support* to a *child in need* rather than that of a child abuse investigator. This family support mindset created a block to communication between her and Abi, preventing the protection of Darren. Patti was very caring towards Abi, but she was not analysing the risk to Darren or investigating allegations of harm. Munro writes of the need for two pairs of glasses, one pair for the role of assessing the child's needs and the other for the role of detective in the investigation of abuse (2003: 170). Importantly, the investigative role includes a focus on targeting the perpetrator and seeking justice for the child. Perceptual screens are highly relevant in this scenario. If Abi's situation is defined by the social worker as that of a well-meaning working-class woman struggling to care for her son, then communication from Abi will be defined as work to improve her parenting skills as the main way of reducing harm to Darren. When it was clearly implied that the injuries were deliberately inflicted, then the hypothesis needed to shift towards Abi or other adults or animals in Darren's life as possibly causing the harm. Abi's communications needed interpretation in the light of that possibility. However, if the situation is defined as one of organized abuse of Darren by the men in the household, with a view to distributing images of the abuse via the internet, Patti might have realized that Abi was also a victim of the network needing urgent protection. In this context, Abi's communications might have been interpreted as a cry for help. All these hypotheses have some validity and needed to be tested through multi-agency co-ordination of information and joint investigation of evidence.

Although asking 'why?' is sometimes given a negative interpretation as implying fault or blame, in the context of critically reflecting on the meaning of communication and the effective transmission of communication, it is important to explore cause and effect linkages (Fook and Askleland 2007: 6). Patti needs to ask why Abi is not prepared to explore how Darren's injuries were caused and continues to divert attention from the issue.

When social workers make judgements about harm to children there is always a risk of either false positives (intervention when it was not required) or false negatives (lack of intervention when it was required). It is always important to ask what the Factor X is in this situation: What can I not see? What have I not been told? What information have I not acquired? Evidence would then need to be sought to prove or disprove the hypothesis formed.

Johari Window

A very useful theory relating to a means of exploring the unknowns within communication is the Johari Window (Luft and Inghram, cited in Lymbery and Postle 2007: 203–204)). This theory provides a model for increasing self-awareness through recognition of differences between our perceptions of ourselves and how others see us. The window consists of four quadrants – in this case relating to Abi and Patti:

1. Information which is known to both Patti and Abi.
2. Information about Patti which Abi can see and knows about but which Patti is unaware of.
3. Information about Patti which Patti knows about but keeps hidden from Abi.
4. Information unknown to both Patti and Abi.

Table 3.1 demonstrates how this model might have been applied and enabled analysis in this case. This would have increased the social worker's reflection on the dynamics of the relationship between herself and the mother and led her to query what evidence Patti may not be aware of. Patti could then have formed hypotheses and begun to test these through evidence gathering by making use of the multi-agency professional network.

Table 3.1 Johari Window

	Known to Patti	Unknown to Patti
Known to Abi	**1 Open**	**2 Unaware**
	Darren is the subject of a child protection plan.	Abi notes Patti is sensitive about not having children herself and not being married.
	Patti is the social worker responsible for making sure the plan is in place.	Abi notes Patti is not assertive and can be manipulated and distracted.
		Abi notes Patti is an inexperienced social worker.
	Patti must co-ordinate the implementation of the plan.	Abi knows that both Declan and Jago live in the household and she hides this from Patti.
	Conclusions have been reached that Abi's explanations do not fit the injuries to Darren.	Abi knows that Darren's injuries are deliberately inflicted by the men in the household and that she has not told Patti.
	Abi does neglect Darren's care.	Abi hasn't told Patti that she is also scared of and at risk from the men who tell her to hide the truth from the social worker to stop her interfering.
	Darren does not have 'easy bruising'.	Abi knows she has deliberately tried to hide new marks from Pattie by covering Darren's face with chocolate.
	Patti is scared of the dog.	Abi knows she has deceived Patti about what the health visitor, family centre worker and other professionals are saying about her parenting.
	Patti suspects the presence of men in the house.	Abi has also deceived Patti about her uncle and father being ill in order to gain Pattie's sympathy.
	Patti does not understand the cause of the injuries to Darren.	Abi knows that she has deliberately made it difficult for Patti and others to see Darren in order that she does not notice the recent injuries.
Unknown to Abi	**3 Hidden**	**4 Unknown**
	Patti does not let Abi know that she is receiving little supervision on the case and feels confused.	Darren's wounds are infected. He is suffering significant harm and is at immediate risk.

Patti does not let Abi know that she has not been trained in child protection work.	Darren's development is impaired. He has become lethargic and no longer cries when hurt – most of the time he sleeps.
Patti does not tell Abi that her manager thinks this case is a family support case even though the protection plan is not working and Abi is not complying with the decisions made.	His developmental stages have not matched with Abi's explanations. Patti's lack of understanding about child development means that she is not sufficiently astute to realize that Darren could not be harming himself as described by Abi.
	Lack of agency co-operation and co-ordination means that neither Patti nor Abi have gained important knowledge about the family composition, the nature of the injuries and sores and details of the neglect and abuse.

Communication: methods

Immediacy

Immediacy is the ability to use the immediate situation to bring about reflection on the communication. It is a way of sharing honestly and openly how the social worker is feeling, thinking and sensing what is being conveyed. It is a powerful method of working which draws attention to what is actually taking place in the 'here and now' and requires the social worker to feel confident in self-reflection. This provides a means of exploring difficulties and removing communication barriers. Patti could have made very good use of this communication method in the above scenarios, for example:

Abi: [*Cries*] They said I hit him. I never hit him. I wouldn't do a thing like that. [*Covers face*] I never hit him. Honestly . . . He hit himself on the fireplace. I'm sure he did.[*Snivels*] That's what Marcia said. It was an accident. Marcia bought me a fireguard.

Patti might have used immediacy to reflect on Abi's non-verbal behaviour, e.g. 'Your explanations do not make sense. They do not explain the injuries. You are obviously very upset at the suggestion that you might have hit Darren. Is that because you feel in some way responsible?' By employing this method Patti is identifying a lack of congruence in Abi's story between her words and her non-verbal behaviour. This opens up the possibility for more meaningful communication and therefore clarification of facts important to the investigation.

Reflective listening

Reflecting listening would have been another effective skill for Patti to use. This refers to carefully listening to another person and repeating back the content enabling correction of any inaccuracies or misunderstandings, essential to evidence collation during an investigation. Reflective listening enables perceptual distortions to be recognized and is a way of checking that the messages sent and received have been understood. For example, when Abi spoke about the place being *a tip* Patti had an opportunity to work with Abi to address the problem. In an investigative approach, Patti might have responded as follows:

Abi: Sorry the place is a bit of a tip. You do think it's a tip don't you? Oh whatever must you think of me? I feel awful. I was going to tidy up. I thought the new social worker is coming this afternoon. I have to tidy up.

Patti: If you are worried about the place being so untidy, and I believe you are, I need you to help me understand why it is in such a mess so that we can sort it out.

Through the reflective listening method, Patti steers the communication forward from Abi's awareness and sense of responsibility towards acting to promote change.

Open questions

Open questions are those that do not suggest a desired response. Using sentences beginning with words such as *tell*, *explain* and *describe*, Pattie would have facilitated Abi in providing more expansive responses contributing to both fact finding and awareness raising in the investigation process. Asking a closed question elicits a yes/no response and does not move the subject on, for example:

Patti: Well we did say, didn't we, that we'd like you to take Darren to see the health visitor?

Abi feels challenged and responds defensively saying that she has been to see the health visitor, when in fact she had not. An open question would have been:

Patti: Tell me how you have been getting on with your visits to the health visitor?

This approach would have been less likely to bring about a negative response although Abi could still have falsified the information. Open questions, in comparison with closed questions, elicit longer and more detailed answers and are less likely to bring about ambiguous and non-verbal responses and more accurate information is likely to be communicated.

Communication: ethics and values

Seeing double

The NSPCC campaign *All Babies Count* emphasizes that babies cannot defend their own rights: 'Early adversity has a long term impact. Pregnancy and the first year are critical. This is a period of rapid development, setting the foundations for all future learning, behaviour and health. Abuse and neglect at this stage may have lifelong consequences' (NSPCC 2011a). Over half of all serious case reviews concern the deaths of children under the age of one year. The main cause of death is neglect but babies suffer all types of harm including sexual abuse. Social workers need to make determined efforts to communicate with babies and pre-verbal children. They should become used to holding babies and playing with them to gain a sense of their well-being (Ferguson 2011: 105). Joint visits with health visitors are an excellent way for social workers to enhance their learning about the normal range of behaviours, as well as the indicators of abuse, in a very young child. A baby may have very rigid posture and muscle tone indicative of a state of tension and mistrust of adults sometimes referred to as *frozen watchfulness*. There may be evidence of neglect such as poor hygiene, severe nappy rash, lack of medical care or low weight gain and there may be physical signs indicative of abuse such as marks or sores. In the Peter Connolly case (see case study below) the social worker noticed that he was banging his head against the cot, seemed to have no response to pain when he fell against the furniture and had sores on his head. Given the difficulties of communication with a baby, it is especially important for social workers to communicate with those who are close to the world of the baby such as nursery staff, health visitors, GPs and, as appropriate, family including any siblings and friends.

The Professional Capability Framework states that social workers should 'recognise that relationships with service users and carers should be based on respect and honesty', but also states 'understand how the means of communication should be modified to address and take account of a range of factors including age, capacity, learning ability and physical ability' (HCPC 2012c: 2.8). The concept of authenticity emphasizes that there should be 'a congruence between what the person says and what she feels and what she does . . . it is the worker's ability to relate to others with personal integrity' (Smale et al. 2000: 204). However, when making judgements about the balance between the rights of a child for protection from harm with the right of the child to a family life (United Nations 1989: Articles 9, 18, 19, 37), there may be ethical dilemmas and authenticity may not always be reflected in communication that is open or straightforward. Social workers need to be able to hold and see simultaneously the needs of the parent and the child. This involves being able to have empathy and concern for the parent, but also to be able to recognize the effects on the child and advocate for them as the most vulnerable member of the family. This is sometimes referred to as the need to *see double*. It can be difficult to reach out to the needs of a parent and to also 'feel connected to the child's powerlessness to protect themselves' (Calder 2008: 69). Feeling empathy, warmth and concern for a parent or carer is fundamental to social work practice and yet this must be situated within a concept of the power differential of the parent/child relationship. Children can remain invisible and undemanding of attention and the social worker must work very hard also to have an authentic response to the child's need for protection. This means proactively reaching out into the world of the child and empathizing with the child's situation. When investigating child abuse, for instance, it is acceptable to communicate with a child without the parent's knowledge if this is in the child's best interest, if the child is likely to be threatened or coerced into silence, if evidence might be destroyed, or if the child does not want the parent involved and is competent to make that decision (DfE 2010: 5.67). It is also acceptable to convene strategy meetings without the parent's knowledge if informing them might place the child at risk of harm (DfE 2010: 5.57).

The strengths model has been promoted for application in a child protection context (Shennan 2006). One example is the Signs of Safety approach developed in Australia (Turnell and Edwards 1997). This aims to promote co-operative relations between families and social workers. The strengths are those factors when the effects counteract the danger and make it less likely to become a reality. Turnell and Edwards underlined that the approach in no way replaced thorough risk assessment in each case and yet this approach, used in the Peter Connolly case, was strongly criticized by the Haringey Serious Case Review:

> The approach has a place in family work and emphasising the strengths of parents is important, but it is not compatible with the authoritative approach to parents in the protective phase of enquiries, assessment and the child protection conference if children are to be protected. When the social worker, their manager, the conference chair and the core group are confident that the parents

> are giving genuine cooperation with the staff, then a family support approach alone like this one is appropriate, as long as there is continued awareness that the assumptions may be mistaken.
>
> (HLSCB 2009: 4.1.24)

A similar view was expressed by Hackett who had concern at strengths-based models in the context of the deletion of the concept of risk within the Assessment Framework (DoH 2000); 'a particular matter of confusion is how much weight should be given to strengths in the face of an identified difficulty and how the mechanisms that operate between, and mediate the relationship amongst, individual risk and protective factors actually work' (Hackett 2003: 169).

Communication: the knowledge base

Professional dangerousness

Knowledge is created through interaction and dialogue in a social and political context. Individual people are researchers of their professional practice in that they must collect and process knowledge in order to act in a meaningful way within their contexts (Fook and Askeland 2007: 9). In this scenario, the social worker specifically needed to be informed about the dynamics of professional dangerousness and to include the environment in which it flourishes, i.e. organizational dangerousness which reflects current political and inter-agency policy agendas (Calder 2008).

Professional dangerousness has been defined as 'the process by which individual workers or multi-disciplinary networks can, mostly unwittingly, act in such a way as to collude with, maintain or increase the dangerous dynamics of the family in which abuse takes place' (Reder et al. 1993). Social workers sometimes make personal allegiances with parents which cloud their professional judgement and objectivity. Patti may have focused on Abi's emotional needs such as depression, unhappy childhood, experience of domestic violence and caring for sick relatives at the expense of recognizing Darren's needs for protection. The policy context of statutory guidance framed Patti's work on the case in her focus on assessment rather than investigation, the strengths model and a family support approach rather than a joint investigation of child abuse and Section 47 protocols (Children Act 1989; DfE 2010).

The *rule of optimism* is particularly relevant in the context of strengths-based practice. The social worker may 'rationalise inaction in respect of child protection needs and on the basis of arguments about the capacities and aspirations of the parents or carers (natural love) and the contextual environment of the child within the family and community (cultural relativism)'

(Calder 2008: 78). In this dynamic of professional dangerousness social workers convince themselves that all is well in the world of the child. Patti was all too willing to believe that Abi was well meaning and genuinely trying her best to look after Darren and this clouded her vision and prevented her focus on the facts about abuse in the case. This was apparent when Patti told Abi she did not need to make observations about the home environment or when she believed the explanation about the caravan door harming his finger.

A knowledge base about the risks of harm to young children would have helped Patti to put her tendency towards optimism in perspective and to understand the prevalence of both neglect and physical harm. For instance, the statistics for child homicide show that two-thirds of children killed by another person are aged under five years. Infants under one are more at risk than older children and in half of all the cases of children killed by another person the parent is the principal suspect (NSPCC 2011c). The NSPCC found that one in nine young adults had suffered severe physical abuse at the hands of an adult which included being hit, kicked, beaten or attacked with a weapon and parents or guardians were responsible for 5.4 per cent of the violent acts (NSPCC 2011b: 8). In a 2009 study of young adults asked to reflect on their childhoods 12 per cent reported parental neglect and a similar number physical abuse (Fisher and Gruescu 2011). Patterns of injury noted over time must be collated and analysed. Reder et al. (1993: 45) noted in their research of serious case reviews that the majority of children 'had been beaten, bruised and sometimes tortured for a long time prior to their deaths. In some instances their injuries had already led to hospital admission.' The numbers of families where there is potentially high risk to babies includes that presented by drug misusing parents, domestic violence, parental alcohol misuse and parents with mental health problems (NSPCC 2011a).

Knowledge about child development would also have enabled Patti to make more perceptive judgements about Darren's well-being. It is impossible for a very young immobile child to cause injuries to themselves. At two to four months Darren would have been rolling over and from about four months old he may also have begun to grab objects. At the ages of six and nine months Darren may or may not have been mobile, although by then he may have been sitting up, crawling and even pulling himself up and climbing and between 11 and 18 months he would have begun walking. Sheridan (2008: 57) provides a detailed knowledge base about children's development including markers of abnormality. There are some specific injuries which should raise alarm bells in relation to young children such as a torn frenulum: 'this can be caused by a direct blow or by force feeding an infant often found in association with other forms of physical abuse' (Barker and Hodes 2007: 34). It is important for a social worker to have a good knowledge about injuries which in a small child are indicative of serious inflicted physical harm. While a toddler might have one bruised eye caused accidentally, repeated bruised eyes or both eyes being bruised are indicative of inflicted injury. Barker and Hodes (2007: 29) refer to suspicious signs being any bruising on a non-ambulant infant, bruising on non-bony prominences such as the trunk, abdomen, cheek, head or ears, any bruising around the mouth, fingertip bruising, slap or punch marks including imprints from a ring or buckle, bruising from bite marks, linear bruising from implements such as sticks and belts, and clusters or patterns of bruising.

When the early injuries were medically assessed as deliberately inflicted, a key consideration would have been Darrens' exact stage of mobility at the time of each injury, unusual marking or infected sores.

The situation in which alleged abuse has occurred must also be explored. It is unusual for a parent to physically harm a passive, sleeping child. There is commonly a trigger such as the child's behaviour being interpreted as in some way challenging to the parent. Abi's comments about Darren's behaviour at the supermarket provide an example of her inability to place his behaviour in a context of his normal developmental stages. Reder and Duncan refer to triggers such as a toileting accident, messy nappy, food refusal or crying which have precipitated violent fatal responses to the child (2003: 69). Family histories are also an important source of knowledge. Parents who have extreme dependency needs themselves may be seeking to meet their own emotional needs through their child and then feel hostility to the child who is unable to perform to their requirements: 'the actual presence of a dependent infant readily awakens their underlying sense of deprivation' (Reder and Duncan 2003: 41). In this scenario Abi explains to Patti the impact of her abusive childhood, and subsequent depression, on her current parenting. A key indicator is her need to feed Darren baby foods despite his age and need for more adult foods (although she denies it). This may mirror her own dependency needs.

The dynamic of parental false compliance

A lesson from serious case reviews has been that practitioners do not listen sufficiently to the child or pay enough attention to their needs. This was because they had focused too much on the parents, especially when the parents were themselves vulnerable. A study of 67 serious case reviews found, that as a consequence, agencies had overlooked the implications for the child. The research provided five main messages regarding children's voices. It stated that children were not seen or heard enough, including by those professionals speaking on their behalf, that parents and carers prevented professionals seeing and listening to children, and where parents were vulnerable their needs were predominant. Finally, agencies did not interpret their findings sufficiently to protect the child (Ofsted 2011: 37). Calder stated that 'parents may be able to convince professionals that they are cooperating to protect the child but in fact a skilled practitioner will be open to considering the possibility of them abusing the child' (2008: 68).

Professionals can become enmeshed with the family and be so collusive that they do not see the needs of the child. Morrison outlined the seven steps of contemplation which is an excellent tool for assisting judgement about parental responses:

> It is too easy to assume, either that clients must be motivated before they walk into the room if change is to happen or conversely to accept a vague promise that they will do whatever we ask as evidence of motivation. It is imperative to distinguish between ambivalence, compliance and change. Some children have suffered because professionals did not distinguish between compliance and change.
>
> (Morrison 1998: 140–141)

The following example provides an analysis of this model in relation to communication in the script:

> *I accept Darren is at risk because he hit himself on the fireplace and he falls on his toys and gets bruises easily*
> At this stage the child will need a protection plan in place because Abi does not accept that the injuries have been confirmed as deliberately inflicted and non-accidental, and dissociates from her parental responsibility to keep Darren safe.

> *I try to stop him but he just keeps hitting his head on the cot. I just don't always get there quick enough.*
> Abi does admit that she is in some way responsible for the neglect but she locates the problem in Darren's behaviour and does not accept responsibility for poor supervision or for the fact that medical opinion states that the injuries are inflicted by an adult. The risk to the child also remains high because Darren's behaviour is defined as problematic by Abi and could prompt an abusive response.

> *I feel bad. Declan is always needing me to help him and there's my uncle and dad who are so sick. I just can't watch Darren all the time. I'm depressed as well, the doctor says so.*
> Abi feels uncomfortable about the alleged abuse. Yet, while evoking some sympathy in the social worker, caution must be taken as this could indicate false compliance as a result of the agency intervention.

I wish it would get sorted so that Darren is more happy. I try and get him to the Family Centre but sometimes he's asleep and I don't like to wake him.
Abi does realize the need for some change and may well comply with some aspects of what the professionals ask, but she still may not acknowledge or understand the requirements of the child protection plan and has little idea of how to achieve the changes needed.

I know I could do better. My friends from the church are going to help me more in caring better for Darren and you and the Family Centre workers are so helpful to me.
Abi has a limited plan for change and shows some motivation. Patti will need to support Abi in making the change.

I don't want my child to be on the list but I realize it will help me get support in working out how to manage Darren better. Next week I'm going to take Darren with me to the Family Centre and the clinic. I know you are checking up on me so I definitely will go. I want him to get better and stop getting all those marks and sores.
The parent realizes they have to make decisions and accept professional support and monitoring. This is a basis for working in partnership with the parent even though Abi is unwilling to acknowledge responsibility.

I'm scared of Declan and Jago. They want me to hide stuff from you and it's too hard. I want to go into a refuge with Darren to keep us both safe.
Abi finally acknowledges that she and Darren are at risk of harm from men in the household. She still does not explain the nature of the risk and is too afraid to speak about what has happened to Darren. However, she wants to be safe and Patti would need to respond immediately to her request before Abi is under further pressure to comply with the abuser's demands.

The key question in this scenario is that the cause of the injuries is unknown and unexplained. There has been no evidence of Abi herself physically harming the child. This has to raise questions about who might have caused the injuries, why she would need to hide this from the social worker and her protective capacity.

Risk assessment of the parent/carer will need to cover five key questions;

1 Is the parent/carer also abusive?
2 Is the parent/carer collusive with the abuser against the interests of the child/children?

3   Can the parent/carer effectively protect the child/children?
4   Can the parent work with professionals to achieve positive change in order to protect the child?
5   What is the child's view of the parent/carer's ability to protect?

Parents and carers cannot be forced into change. Rushing may increase their sense of failure and low self-esteem, leading to defensiveness and non-compliance. The investigation must focus on enhancing the parent's motivation to change. However, the child needs to develop and grow in a safe environment and their timescales may not be the same as those of the parent. It is a matter of judgement how long professionals should wait for a parent to change when a child is meanwhile experiencing abuse. In decision-making, the type of abuse, the age of the child and the potential for change must be evaluated by a multi-agency team and clearly reflected in the outline of objectives to be achieved within decision-making and planning processes.

Reder et al. (1993) noted that social workers often had no useful method of collating information in order to make a meaningful analysis. A relatively simple way to structure information is to create a chronology. This may be a full account of every detail of the case or a more selective list of allegations and incidents of abuse and the outcomes of Section 47 (Children Act 1989) investigation. These methods enable the social worker to consider the case in perspective over time and to realize that a recent incident must be analysed in the context of previous incidents and investigations. These chronologies also enable analysis of the decrease or escalation of incidents and levels of risk and comparison of parental explanations over time as well as providing substantial evidence in the event of court proceedings (see Table 3.2).

Organizational dangerousness

Patti should have been working within a joint investigation team, in compliance with Section 47 (Children Act 1989) which states the statutory duty to investigate where there is reasonable cause to suspect actual or likely significant harm to a child. She should have been working to the decisions of multi-agency strategy meetings as required in the statutory guidance *Working Together* (DfE 2010). In this process social workers take the lead working jointly with police and other agencies. However, by recommending that police focus solely on the investigation of crime, Laming, in the Victoria Climbié Inquiry report, effectively removed police from joint work with social workers in the majority of child abuse referrals where, at the initial stages, crime may not be evident (2003: 14.57). Police child abuse teams were reduced and strategy meetings, the main statutory forum for police, social workers, doctors, teachers and other professionals to plan an investigation were largely replaced with strategy discussions by telephone between police

Table 3.2 Child protection case chronology

Date/time	Source	Key events	Information	Health	Carer's view	Child's view	Professional comment
24.10.2012 2.30 pm	Health visitor records.	Abi and Darren visit clinic.	Concern at Darren being very tired and unresponsive.	There is some weight loss which is of concern.	Abi says Darren has had a cold and lost his appetite even though she made him his favourite foods.		Appointment made for next week to monitor weight loss. Informed social worker.
25.10.2012 10.00 am	Children's services records.	Family centre worker left message.	Abi arrived at parenting class without Darren. Fourth time she has done this. Since the conference she has only brought him twice.		Abi says Darren is asleep at that time of day and she is reluctant to disturb him.		Told Abi that the social worker would be informed that the child protection plan is not being implemented as agreed.
3.1.2013 3.00 pm	Children's services records.	Home visit. Abi and Darren have been missing. Address unknown.	Abi says they were staying with her uncle who is sick. She did not realize she had to inform Patti as part of the child protection plan.	Darren is pale and listless. He has a bandage on his finger. He has sores on his face and skin irritation. Doctor has provided antibiotic cream.	Injury caused by catching finger in caravan door. Sores are caused through Darren scratching himself.		Appointment made with child protection doctor to consider comparison of injuries and marks with previous inflicted injuries and to advise joint investigation about the nature of current injuries and marks. Doctor to liaise with GP and health visitor. Photographs to be taken of injuries.

Source: Davies and Duckett (2008: 28).

Table 3.3 Incident chart

Date	Allegation /incident	Carer explanation	Action taken	Outcome for the child
1.2.2012 1.00 pm	Abi says she leaves Darren in the cot for extended periods.	This is because she cannot manage Darren while she is shopping.	Patti informed Abi that this is unacceptable and places Darren at risk of harm. Information shared at strategy meeting.	Child protection plan includes requirement that Abi must not leave Darren in his cot in the house on his own. Family centre staff to discuss with Abi strategies for managing Darren while shopping.

Developed from Calder and Hackett (2003: 127).

and social workers. This has created a situation of organizational dangerous-ness as while police focus on crime and social workers conduct assessments of need, the joint investigation of child abuse has been minimized leaving a gap in protection systems.

Professional non-compliance with procedures is a key aspect of profes-sional dangerousness and yet this must be analysed in the context of organi-zational dangerousness. *Working Together* stated that the core assessment 'is the means by which a Section 47 enquiry is carried out' (DfES 2006: 5.60; DfE 2010: 5.62). This is inaccurate. Assessment informs the Section 47 investiga-tion but as a single process will not provide a child with protection from abuse. Assessments require parental consent for interviewing or medically examining the child and for making agency checks whereas this is not the case in an investigation. Also the assessment has to be conducted to strict timescales whereas an investigative process cannot be time limited (Calder and Hackett 2003).

In this scenario Patti was conducting an assessment in isolation from stat-utory processes and joint work with police. Additionally, there was no context of strategy meetings and investigative techniques such as profiling the abusers, collating intelligence, examining the scene of the alleged crimes, forensic anal-ysis of the injuries and witness evidence. The focus was solely on Abi's parenting capacity in the context of Patti's assumption that Abi was prioritizing Darren's best interests. In this respect Patti reflected national trends where, particularly since the abolition of the child protection register in 2008, child protection plans have become based mainly on assessment rather than investigation processes. Assessment is the wrong tool because investigation cannot be time limited or based on mechanistic questions. Joint investigation demands skilled evaluation of child interviews, forensic and medical evidence, adult accounts and knowledge about perpetrators. No two cases are the same and the complex-ities are immense. Since the abolition of the register, alarm bells no longer ring with the emergency services and strategy meetings have given way to telephone calls to police often to confirm that social workers must go it alone. Without ongoing joint work with police, social workers alone cannot achieve the task of protection, and a lack of investigation leads to faulty decisions – not only abused children being missed but families wrongly accused.

Burke (1994: 19) refers to the *invisible man syndrome* where the impact of the man's actions are seen but he remains invisible. How then might Patti have discovered the role of the men in Abi's household? In the absence of formal child protection processes, Patti did not co-ordinate reports from the health visitor, family centre or police and this left a gap in information which Abi inaccurately filled. This led to some role confusion and poor co-ordination between the agencies working in the case. For example, Patti received information about the address of a man in the household but did not report this to the police and she accepted the health visitor's assessment as conveyed by Abi. There may have been other adults in Darren's world who had knowledge about his care such as friends from the church and Patti could have spoken with them. The exaggeration of hierarchy is another aspect of professional dangerousness where people of low status who often are close to and have knowledge of the child such as neighbours and childminders are excluded from being sources to inform the professional network. A strategy meeting could have planned this approach as part of the investigation in clarifying what was known about Darren and his safety.

Abi avoided contact with professionals. This is the dynamic of closure where the parent shuts out professional involvement and appointments are missed, curtains closed and doors locked. In this case Abi went away without disclosing her and Darren's whereabouts. Reder and Duncan found that 'it was evident that episodes of closure had coincided with periods of escalating abuse and also tended to lead up to the death of the child' (2003: 129). Awareness of avoidance and closure should precipitate a multi-agency strategy to put in place child protection plans to ensure that the family are within professional monitoring.

A key aspect of organizational dangerousness is whether the workplace is a safe working environment for the social worker. Reder et al. stated:

> Many factors contribute to a secure setting, including adequate training, regular supervision and support, clear procedural guidelines, adequate funding and staffing, low staff turnover, an optimal caseload, continuity in management, a stable organisational structure, good secretarial backup, requisite facilities and so on. All these elements combine to provide the mechanical means for effective communication and also a context within which the workers feel valued, respected and supported
>
> (1993: 69)

Patti was inexperienced and untrained in child protection. She also received little supervision on the case.

CASE STUDY AND REFLECTION

Investigation in the Peter Connolly case

There are many comparisons to be made between the case of Darren and that of Peter Connolly. There are also some differences. This case study reflects the shortcomings of the investigative processes in Peter's story and emphasizes the importance of professional compliance with statutory guidance.

Peter Connolly died on the 3 August 2007 aged 17 months. He had bruising to his body, a tooth missing, a torn frenulum and marks to his head. A post-mortem revealed further injuries such as a tooth which was found in his colon, eight fractured ribs and a fractured spine. He had been living with his mother Tracey Connolly and his siblings, her boyfriend Stephen Barker, his brother Jason Owen, Owen's 'girlfriend' aged 15, and Owen's own children. Following the trial in 2008 all three adults were acquitted of murder. The mother admitted causing or allowing the death of a child and the two men were convicted of the same offence.

From the age of about nine months, Peter's mother provided professionals with inconsistent explanations for serious injuries including that the dog had caused scratches, that Peter had fallen on his toys and harmed himself through his own behaviours such as head banging. She did not inform social workers about adults living in the household, although she did mention this to other professionals and support workers. As there was no ongoing Section 47 investigation, these facts were often unreported or uncollated so that there was no risk assessment of the men in the home. It may have been that she was also at risk of harm from these men and covered up facts to protect herself. She appeared to, but in fact did not, comply with the protection plan and, with hindsight, it is clear that she avoided professional contact when Peter had new injuries. She missed appointments and played one professional off against another. Despite paediatric opinion stating that Peter's injuries were inflicted and reports of neglect such as severe nappy rash, head lice, weight loss and unattended infected sores, the professional response was to provide family support services and *concrete solutions* which were practical provisions such as a fireguard and sofa. Some of the later injuries were very unusual such as torn and missing fingernails. The serious case review drew attention to the dynamic of false compliance in the case. The following excerpts from the review provide an opportunity to make comparisons with the dynamics outlined in the scenario about Darren and Abi:

Although perhaps not consciously, a parent/carer in the mother's situation is testing the resolve of the safeguarding and child protection
systems. She had not yet found it necessary to disclose what has
happened to Peter, and in particular who had caused the injuries. From
the beginning she was given every indication that she may not need to
do so.

(HLSCB 2009: 4.1.2)

Agencies were too willing to believe the mother's accounts of herself,
her care of the children, the composition of her household, and the
nature of her friendship network . . . The danger is an over-identification
with the service user in a wish to support and protect the child's place in
the family. There was already reason to believe that she was not being
truthful about the injuries to her child.

(HLSCB 2009: 4.1.3)

Peter was the subject of a child protection conference in December
2006, with injuries so serious that they met the threshold for care
proceedings. Although it cannot be known for certain how the injuries
occurred, the medical view of the causes of the injuries went as far as it
could in offering a non-accidental opinion – and it was gradually
discounted. The likely explanation is that the injuries were not regarded
as sufficiently serious and that there was an over-identification with the
parent whose account of possible explanations was perceived to be
plausible.

(HLSCB 2009: 4.1.4)

What was required was an authoritative approach to the family, with a
very tight grip on the intervention. Ms A needed to be challenged and
confronted about her poor parenting and generally neglectful approach
to the home . . . The passive acceptance of her continued poor parenting
was a fundamental problem in the inter-agency approach.

(HLSCB 2009: 4.1.12)

The Serious Case Review was critical of the *family support* intervention calling
for an authoritarian approach: 'it never was established that there was a basis to
work in a family support model with Mrs A. The use of this model was assumed
to be self-evident from the beginning' (HLSCB 2009: 4.1.20). When Peter's social
worker was asked during the criminal trial about her role in the case, she responded
that she had been there to support the family and when Haringey Local
Safeguarding Children's Board responded to the media initially they presented a
document entitled 'Support Offered to Family of Child A' (HLSCB 2008). It is

significant that neither described work to protect Peter. Although Peter's name was on the child protection register, the child protection plan was one of family support provision, such as parenting programmes and practical help, rather than ongoing investigation of identified significant harm. The social workers utilized the *signs of safety* strengths model which was said to have influenced the family support progress of the case (HLSCB 2008: 4.1.23).

Following the Peter Connolly case, Ofsted (2008) reported that 'social care, health and police authorities do not communicate and collaborate routinely and consistently to ensure effective assessment, planning and review of cases of vulnerable children . . . too often assessments fail to identify those who are at immediate risk of harm and address their needs'. It was later found that 60 cases at 'extreme risk' had been ignored and front-line workers had not visited the children's homes to check on their safety (Singh 2009). In the Peter Connolly case, the police focus was on the investigation of crime and the social work focus was mainly on the assessment of need and completion of the assessment form. The joint investigation of child abuse did not take place effectively through the application of appropriate procedures. The child protection register had not been abolished in 2007, but its role was already being undermined. Key professionals did not attend the conferences which were not adequately informed by investigation, unexplained injuries had not been investigated in a forensic way and the possible abusers had not been identified. The police role was limited as they did not follow through a detailed investigative role with social workers or regularly progress the findings through strategy meetings. Core group meetings held after the child protection conference were the main planning forum, but failed to initiate the convening of strategy meetings as new concerns became evident. The core group meetings were chaired by the social worker who had no child protection training and police and paediatricians did not attend. Agencies which did attend were the health visitor and parenting class workers working within the family support model. Ofsted commented that attendance at core group meetings was variable and this 'limited the opportunities for ensuring that the child protection plan was on track' (Ofsted 2008: 10). When Peter had further unexplained marks and injuries he was sent to the child development clinic rather than a named safeguarding nurse or child protection doctor who should have been monitoring his injuries throughout.

A lack of compliance with child protection procedures led to no proper forum for the communication and collation of information from all agencies. For example, the parenting programme staff 'did not share information about Baby P's family situation with any other agencies or NHS trusts despite this information having significant implications for the care of Baby P within the family house' (CQC 2009: 17). There was no arrangement to inform the social worker if the mother did not attend and if Peter was not with her. She went to nine out of thirteen sessions and took Peter to only four (HLSCB 2008: 4.2.1). As part of the family support approach both the parenting programme and the housing support agency held very important information about the family but this was not shared within the strategy meeting, child protection conference or core groups. Some of this information related to men in the household. Background information should have brought to the attention of police and social workers that a relative of the mother had been a central victim in the Islington child abuse case. This would have alerted professionals to the need to examine possible networks of abuse which might have been abusing the child in a context of organized abuse (Fairweather 2008a, 2008b). Further details relating to the case may be found in Davies (2008a, 2008b, 2009).

All points outlined above underscore the extent to which complex and essential communication strategies must be central to investigating child abuse.

Questions to aid reflection

Drawing on the knowledge presented in this chapter, and your learning from analysis of the script, consider the many layers of communication breakdown in the Peter Connolly case and specifically address the following questions:

 How might the social workers have communicated better with the children?

 How did a collusive social work approach with the mother lead to a lack of focus on other perpetrators in these cases?

 How did the conflation of assessment and investigation affect communication in these cases?

 Did a police focus on crime distract them from communication with social workers about significant harm?

 Why was there no effective Section 47 strategy in place to protect the child and focus on the abusers?

 How did the use of core group rather than strategy meetings negatively affect communication between child protection professionals?

 How did the application of the family support model of social work distract social workers and police from their core task of protecting vulnerable abused children?

Agencies and websites

Social workers need to be informed about the key agencies involved in this area of work so that they know where to access specialist advice and support.

Association of Child Abuse Lawyers (ACAL). Practical support for UK lawyers and other professionals working for adults and children who have been abused. www.childabuselawyers.com

Children are Unbeatable Alliance. A broad-based UK alliance promoting children's right to be protected from all corporal punishment. www.childrenareunbeatable.org.uk

Children's Rights Alliance for England (CRAE). Seeks the full implementation of the Convention on the Rights of the Child in England. www.crae.org.uk

London Safeguarding Children Board (LSCB). Provides advice and support to London's 32 Local Safeguarding Children Boards (LSCBs). www.londonscb.gov.uk

National Association of People Abused in Childhood (NAPAC). A registered charity providing support and a helpline to people abused in childhood. www.napac.org.uk

National Society for the Prevention of Cruelty to Children (NSPCC). The NSPCC Inform website provides up-to-date research findings and statistics relating to child protection. www.nspcc/inform

Recommended reading

Calder, M. (2008) Professional dangerousness. Causes and contemporary features, in M. Calder (ed.) *Contemporary Risk Assessment in Safeguarding Children*. Lyme Reg's: Russell House.

Davies, L. and Duckett, N. (2008) *Proactive Child Protection and Social Work*. Exeter: Learning Matters.

Reder, P., Duncan, S. and Gray, M. (2003) *Beyond Blame: Child Abuse Tragedies Revisited*. London: Routledge.

Saunders, B. and Goddard, C. (2010) *Physical Punishment in Childhood: The Rights of the Child*. Chichester: Wiley.

4 Use of power: Representing the best interests of an unaccompanied asylum seeking young person

Introduction

Chapter content

The nature, scope and dimension of power as applied in social work communication will determine the quality of relationships and the impact of interventions. Power has the potential to be used and interpreted in many different ways. Its use and authority within social work protects children and is a means of challenging oppression, inequalities and discrimination at every level. The dominant social work discourse has defined power negatively as a tool of social oppression and the use of power by social workers has gained an unpopular image linked with concepts of social control and being an agent of the state. Okitikpi (2011) presents a different view, examining the responsible use of power in achieving social justice for young people. It is important to differentiate between *power over* which is the capacity to exert force be it physical, intellectual or structural, and *power to* or *power with* which are egalitarian concepts emphasizing the ability of social workers to influence and make positive change (Tew 2006; Thorpe 2011: 85).

In the context of immigration policies and social work with a young person, the use of power in this chapter is interrogated to demonstrate building, confirming and enabling while fully comprehending the misuse of its authority to collude, constrain and control. Without a comprehensive understanding of these complex processes, and critical reflection on their professional and agency role, social workers risk contributing further to the young person's marginalization and oppression. They need to define themselves as having an ability to influence situations and to think beyond classifying the young people as entirely helpless in the face of extraordinary difficulties and human rights violations.

This chapter focuses on social work with an unaccompanied asylum seeking child (UASC). This is a child under the age of 18 who is not living with their parent, relative or guardian in the UK and needs the care and protection of welfare services in the country of asylum while their claim is examined and settled. In most cases these young people become referred to social workers by the UK Border Agency (UKBA) at ports of entry after they have made long and frightening journeys from their home countries and experienced intimidating and often abusive UK immigration processes. It is very difficult for a social worker to enter the world of the child in this situation and to do so they must have knowledge about the complexity of the child's traumatic experience, refrain from making assumptions and be open to hearing their accounts. Kohli refers to the silence of young people who want to face the present first, the future next and the past last (2006: 208). The social worker must also be a strong advocate for the rights of young people within an oppressive and discriminatory social and legal context. A young person's account of his journey and experience of being an unaccompanied asylum seeking child is included as the case study.

Summary of the script

For the purpose of demonstrating the enabling and appropriate use of power in social work to support and represent the interests of a UASC, three dialogues are provided. In the first, the allocated social worker, Magda, visits a young person, Jahandar, following an incident of self-harm. She must assess the situation, including his safety and well-being. It is crucial that she connects and relates sufficiently with the young person in order to understand his needs and to advocate for him. However, in the first dialogue Magda struggles to engage with Jahandar which is in part the result of a lack of knowledge and understanding of his background and past experiences. The second dialogue, presented as a supervision session between Magda and her manager, addresses the practice shortcomings demonstrated in dialogue one. The third is an alternative dialogue between Magda and Jahandar in which Magda relates more meaningfully to him using advice and direction from supervision. This results in an improved communication between them and informs Magda's report to the resources panel.

The script: the social worker, Magda, communicates with an unaccompanied asylum seeking boy, Jahandar, in order to fully represent his views to a resources panel

Setting the scene

Jahandar is an unaccompanied young person aged 16 years. He is 5´10" of slim build and is a practising Muslim from Afghanistan. He identifies his ethnicity as Pashtun with Pashtu as his first language. He is a quiet young man choosing to engage only with those he has developed a relationship with and even then these relations tend to be more functional than friendly. Professionals describe him as polite and compliant, and one report refers to his winning smile. He likes football but his shy demeanour has not endeared him to team mates and he is often seen returning from football practice alone. In the 16 months since his arrival in the UK he has established a competent command of English. His school head of year is very pleased with his progress and he has good physical health.

Jahandar's social worker, Magda, works in the looked after children's team. She came to the UK three years ago from Poland where she was employed for several years as a children's social worker. Jahandar has been in his current foster placement for the past nine months and has been allocated to Magda for most of that time. Two younger children, siblings, are also placed there. Magda has become increasingly aware of Jahandar's discontent and following recent visits has expressed her worry about his emotional well-being. He has told her that he doesn't sleep very well, he seems disinterested when discussing plans and has become monosyllabic in his responses. Although never particularly talkative, this is a change. She has also begun to experience recent visits as frustrating and worrying but his foster carer is quick to reassure her that all is well. Jahandar is a lovely boy, she says, a little quiet, keeps himself to himself but he is no trouble at all.

First dialogue

A referral has been received from the out-of-hours team which responded to an emergency on Saturday. Jahandar cut his arms quite badly. The attending general practitioner (GP) described the cuts as superficial and Jahandar as not in physical danger, although he is worried about his mental well-being and has made a referral to the child and adolescent mental health service (CAMHS).

Jahandar returned home with the foster carer but refused to discuss or explain what happened. A younger child in the placement alerted Monica, the foster carer, on Saturday when he went into Jahandar's room and found him using a razor blade to cut his arm. The child was shocked and upset.

On receipt of the referral on Monday morning and, after a very brief conversation with her team manager, the allocated social worker, Magda, goes immediately to the foster home to visit Jahandar and to complete an assessment.

Comment

Magda is worried about Jahandar but also concerned about an appointment she had to rearrange in order to make this visit. She does not like changing arrangements at the last minute and the children she was due to see will be upset. She is thinking about how she will make it up to them.

The social worker arrives, and at the foster carer's suggestion, the visit takes place in the family living room.

Comment

Visits to young people are best conducted in spaces identified by them. The choice may even indicate the nature or content of the conversation they might wish to have. Taking direction from a young person allows them some control in the process and respects them as participants.

Magda: Hi Jahandar. I am pleased to see you. How are you?

Jahandar: Hi. [*Looks at the social worker briefly with a nervous smile and then looks away*]

Magda: [*Sits in an armchair opposite Jahandar*] So, are you able to tell me what happened Jahandar? I was very worried when I heard this morning about the incident.

Comment

Here Magda asks a closed question allowing only a yes/no response. She could reframe the question as 'Tell me what happened' or 'I'd really like you to help me understand what happened. Please tell me about it.'

Jahandar: [*Changes position on the sofa, pulls at the sleeves of his jumper*] Why am I not able to go to school today? I want to go to school.

Magda: I'm afraid the doctor advised Monica to keep you at home. I guess he thought school might be a bit much after what happened. But it's given me the opportunity to talk to you so that's good! Can we talk about what happened? I know it's difficult, but I want to know what's going on.

Jahandar: [*Long silence*] It's nothing, just . . .

Magda: It's definitely not nothing. You cut your arms and we are all very concerned.

Jahandar: [*Remains silent*]

Comment

Still preoccupied by a time constraint, worried about Jahandar, and driven by a genuine need to understand what happened and why, Magda struggles to set up meaningful communication and resorts to quick-fired multiple questions that place her, rather than Jahandar, at the centre and make it difficult for him to respond. Questions beginning with 'Can you' or 'Would you' invite a yes/no response. It would have been better to say 'Let's have a talk about what happened.' Paralanguage is used to describe the way that words are communicated such as the tone of voice which might be gentle, harsh, excitable or dull. It includes the speed of communication and the loudness or softness. The difference between what is said and how it is said often acts as a communication barrier (Thompson 2011: 101). Here Magda's paralanguage creates a communication block as her tone denotes frustration with his lack of response.

Magda: Did something happen at school? That's what Monica thinks. Has she spoken to you about it? Did someone say something or do something that upset you Jahandar?

Jahandar: No [*Looking down*]. I don't know why I did it. Can I get a drink?

Magda: Yes of course, I could do with a drink myself. But we do need to talk about how you are feeling and if you are unhappy. I have to review your plan and report back to my manager about what's happening.

Jahandar: [*Alarmed, looks back at Magda on his way to get the drinks*] What does that mean? What are they going to do? I was just messing around, I know it was a stupid thing to do. What is your manager going to do? It didn't mean anything.

Comment

Jahandar thinks he is being blamed for his self-harming behaviour and becomes anxious and defensive. Magda is relieved Jahandar has replied with more than one word but she has little awareness of the anxiety she has created or of the new barrier to communication which has resulted. Being open with him about the responsibility of the work can be transparent and empowering, but timing and appropriateness to the situation as well as context are crucial to guard against fear and alienation for the young person.

Magda: Well let's talk a little bit about it so I can decide if anything needs to happen and maybe nothing needs to happen, but I have to assess it. We are not angry with you Jahandar, just worried.
[*They return with drinks from the kitchen.*]
Magda: I need to make a quick call to the office. It's very busy on a Monday morning and I had to pass another appointment on to a colleague. But that's fine I want to be here. I want to be sure we get it right for you.

Comment

This is a mixed message to Jahandar about his social worker's priorities, and attention is again directed away from his situation.

Jahandar: OK.
[*Magda returns to the living room having made the call.*]
Magda: So, where were we? Can you tell me anything at all about what you were feeling on Saturday?
Jahandar: I spoke to the doctor. I told him I'm OK. I don't know why I did it. I don't want to live here anymore. [*Looks very upset*]
Magda: But I thought you were happy here. Can you tell me what's changed? Where would you like to go? It might not be that easy.

Comment

While professionally realistic, suggesting a barrier/problem at this stage, at the moment of a possible break-through, is likely to discourage a distraught Jahandar from communicating. Magda makes assumptions rather than supporting Jahandar in providing his own account as he feels ready to do so.

Jahandar: I don't know, I don't know. Can I go to my room now?
Magda: Yes of course, I'm sorry you are upset. I am going to try and work this out. I do want to help you. I'll come back later in the week. Maybe you will feel more like talking then. OK?
Jahandar: OK.

Comment

Magda needed to have an understanding of self-harm in order to realize why Jahandar might be reticent to communicate with her about what happened. Young people are ambivalent about the behaviour and often ask for recognition and acceptance of it as a valid way of expressing distress. They are also embarrassed to speak about it, often remaining silent (Spandler 1996: 112). Reasons for self-harm include 'not having to think about painful and preoccupying memories, thoughts or worries, getting out of a difficult situation for a while and creating a situation of comfort and security like a *haven in a heartless world*' (Spandler 1996: 26).

Second dialogue

It is the following day and the social worker is having her fortnightly supervision with her manager. They discuss her work with Jahandar.

Supervisor: OK, let's look at your cases. Can you bring me up to date on Jahandar, your assessment from yesterday and let's see if we need to review his plan and placement. I thought things were going OK at Monica's.

Magda: Yes, we all thought things were going relatively OK though I had noticed he was more withdrawn and quiet recently. Maybe we should have anticipated something like this.

Supervisor: It is often the case that the least demanding cases drift with problems just below the radar. Was there any psychological support identified in his plan? I seem to remember his assessment identifying concerns about how little Jahandar had been able to tell us about life before he came here.

Magda: We have been waiting for a space at the Young Refugees Project for peer support and he has a mentor at school. As far as I know he remains reticent about his past. He has said very little to Monica. I thought we had a reasonably good relationship but he was so sad and anxious yesterday and I couldn't get much from him. I felt really bad leaving without having established exactly what the problem is. The CAMHS team will fast track his referral due to the self-harm incident. I've made his head of year aware at school, and the GP is satisfied so long as Jahandar's situation is monitored closely while we're waiting for the CAMHS assessment. I informed the Independent Reviewing Officer and we have arranged to bring forward the Looked After Children review.

Supervisor: Good. You have done well to put all that in place. I know how busy you are with your other cases and am aware of the emotional impact. If we make sure we have addressed the critical things first, then how you are feeling and finish with moving forward with the case. How about that?

Magda: Yes that's OK.

Supervisor: You need to make sure everything is accurately recorded, including your analysis of the situation based on your ongoing work with Jahandar including information from the network. Don't forget to let the child protection team know, given the nature of the incident. You may not have had time to think of this but it is also important to speak to the social worker for the child who discovered Jahandar with the razor. This must have been very difficult for that child and it will need to be addressed. Make sure you record that you have done this. How is Jahandar at the reviews? Is he able to contribute, meaningfully I mean, in terms of what he wants?

Magda: Well, he pretty much leaves it to me but he does respond to questions, especially from the Independent Reviewing Officer (IRO). They have a good relationship.

Supervisor: That is helpful because a change in plan, especially if it requires extra resources, will need the full support of the IRO. OK, let's talk about your visit yesterday.

Magda describes the visit; Jahandar's reluctance to share, his emotional presentation and her overall impression of the meeting not being productive or worth while.

Supervisor: Sounds like you did most of the talking, but it is often the way we respond to reticence in others, especially if there is a crisis. Silence is OK you know, it doesn't have to be oppressive. For children and young people, being easy with their silence can be supportive, and reassuring. Even when they are ready to tell their story, it is important that they trust it can be heard.

Magda: But how do we get to know and understand what is going on? The consequences are enormous if we don't know.

Supervisor: Jahandar knows you are an important person in his life. He is aware that you can do things for him but he is also very likely to be wary or frightened of your power. His reaction when you said you would be discussing the situation with me, for instance, was very telling.

Magda: He did say that he didn't want to live at Monica's any more, but I'm not sure if he really means that. She has no problems with him and has the impression that he is generally fine.

Supervisor: Being undemanding and easy to have around is not necessarily an indicator of being satisfied and content. It seems to me that you need to reassure Jahandar that he can trust you, and that this incident has not changed your regard for him or your commitment to helping him. It is hard to see positives when we are worried

Magda acknowledges her feelings and how she hasn't been able to concentrate properly on her other cases since she visited Jahandar. She has been thinking a lot about it at home and she got very little sleep last night. She worries about Jahandar self-harming again.

Magda: I can't help thinking that we haven't really helped Jahandar. What he must have been through in order to get here, we have no idea. He seems so sad and isolated and now this.

Supervisor: It seems to me that you have established empathy. It is likely he will have picked this up (without being able to articulate it), and that will be the basis for building more trust. Jahandar's self-harm incident is an indicator of how he is feeling, a coping strategy. We also know that children who have had adverse experiences struggle psychologically and have difficulty communicating. Feeling as uncertain as you do about how to help is not unusual.

Magda: Just as well the CAMHS team will be carrying out their assessment soon; otherwise I would feel really lost with this.

Supervisor: You mustn't underestimate your role here or your relationship with Jahandar. You are key to creating the plan that emerges and your recommendations must be based on his wishes and feelings.

Magda: What are the options for him?

Supervisor: In the first instance it is important to get some sense of what he wants, even if that proves difficult. If we have options identified for him and share those, chances are that's what will become the focus of the meeting and Jahandar may not see a reason then to participate especially if he doesn't agree.

Magda: I'll visit him again next week and hopefully I'll have more luck.

Supervisor: We can't rely on luck. Jahandar can't rely on luck. I want you to visit him again before the end of this week and make time to follow that up with another the following week as it is going to take more time. Sensitive persistence can be very rewarding. If Jahandar knows you are prioritizing him and making space and time without crowding him, he is more likely to see you as an advocate, someone he can trust. That's what we want isn't it?

Magda: Yes, of course but already I have had to put other tasks and cases aside for this case – what about them?

Supervisor: Let's not think about that for the moment and stay concentrated on Jahandar. We will look at your impending tasks before we finish. Let's think of models of direct work that can help to engage a reluctant, worried young person.

Magda: I have an idea about adapting the Three Houses Model (Weld 2009). It can be used for planning as well as assessment and ensures the voice of the young person is central.

Supervisor: Sounds good. If you can apply it so that Jahandar feels it is a shared process, that is, his input is valued, his wishes are taken seriously, you are not afraid to address the self-harm incident in the context of his safety, and you help him develop strategies you can both take responsibility for implementing in the immediate future. If he can believe in this process he is more likely to tell you what might work for him. If you are invested in the plan that emerges, it is more likely to be meaningful and therefore actioned. He may even begin to refer to his past – but that's not what we're looking for right now so should it come up, give him time to speak, listen, show interest and compassion, but don't let yourself be drawn into any form of interrogation of his story.

Magda: Sounds too good to be true, like as if anything is possible. What if I can't make it happen? He may not even talk with me.

Supervisor: The more inclusive you are, in your communication and approach as well as your method, the more likely he will be to engage. A strengths-based approach without neglecting the risk may provide new possibilities.

Magda: Yes, that is the basis of the model.

Supervisor: Like I said earlier you are committed to helping Jahandar and have known him for some time – that's a good starting point for this piece of work. You also have a good idea of what is unrealistic and if you are unsure do come back to me. Let Jahandar know from the outset that you will be putting all plans past your manager, and to start with think broadly and creatively.

Magda: OK. We have a team meeting next Monday. Maybe I could bring this case for discussion. More ideas may be generated that I can use.

Supervisor: Don't forget to factor in Jahandar's adolescence and the importance of his identity. No doubt that will be taken up by CAMHS, but it must also inform your analysis. Sometimes we over-read silences and particularly with unaccompanied asylum seekers maybe we tend to pathologize, though because he has self-harmed we clearly need to be careful. But equally we don't want to neglect the ordinary or expected moods of teenagers.

Magda: I will arrange a visit for Thursday after football, though maybe he won't go this week after what happened. Yes, it feels more concrete now, like I might have a way in. Perhaps if we are involved in an activity like the adapted model, Jahandar may find it less intense and easier to express himself.

Supervisor: Yes, definitely. Keep me informed.

Supervision on Jahandar's case concludes.

Comment

In this scenario the supervisor recognizes and acknowledges the emotional impact of Jahandar's self-harming and skilfully uses the care and concern expressed by Magda to identify empathy as a communication method to underpin her direct work. Through reflection on emotional responses, social workers can rework how they see themselves and others. As applied here, Magda gains an increased sense of personal agency, has less anxiety and is better able to use her power to promote Jahandar's interests.

While encouraging a therapeutic style of social work practice, the supervisor helps Magda to think about Jahandar's practical world as well as being alert to risk. Using this approach to casework supervision, Magda gets emotional support, practical advice, clear instruction and a working through of the issues in Jahandar's case such as to experience a shared process that she can model with him.

Alternative dialogue

The following dialogue provides an example of good communication between Magda and Jahandar. Consider the following points as a guide to good practice:

- the importance of Magda's learning from supervision
- the change in Magda's communication approach
- how Jahandar is better supported and enabled to communicate
- Magda's positive use of power in advocating for and representing Jahandar's wishes.

Third dialogue

Following a phone conversation between Jahandar and Magda, a visit will take place on Friday after football practice, which it seems Jahandar does want to go to. On the phone he appears initially disinterested in another visit but does not object.

All the other agencies involved have been made aware of the incident at the weekend and the school nurse, who agreed with the GP to check on Jahandar, has reported no concerns, although she said he was embarrassed when she checked his arms and asked him a few questions.

Magda arrives at the foster carers' but Jahandar has not yet returned from football. While waiting she speaks with Monica and establishes that Jahandar has not mentioned the self-harm incident and has been spending less and less time with the family. He tends to retreat to his bedroom. However, Jahandar did speak to Sam who witnessed the incident. He apologized to Sam for the upset and played computer games with him that evening. This was unusual and unsolicited by the foster carer.

Jahandar arrives. He doesn't mind where the visit takes place. Magda suggests that they go to the nearby community centre where there is a quiet room and they can pick up some takeaway food on route.

While driving to the community centre.

Magda: So, how have you been Jahandar?

Jahandar: Fine.

Magda: I was pleased to hear you went to football today and Monica says you have been fine since the weekend, although you've been very quiet.

Jahandar: Not much to say. Everyone is always wanting to talk. What's there to talk about?

Magda: Monica said you were very kind to Sam. That's good Jahandar. It's not easy to think about others when you're having a bad time yourself. It shows you have a lot of understanding.

Jahandar: Sam's OK. He's annoying sometimes and I don't want him coming into my room.

Magda: I appreciate that. It can be irritating having to put up with younger kids when you are a teenager, but it was lucky for us that Sam went into your room when he did, otherwise we wouldn't have known you were worried and upset.

[*Jahandar shifts uneasily and looks out of the passenger window.*]

Magda: Do you like cars Jahandar?

Jahandar: Yeh, course. Can't wait to learn to drive. Just take off. This car's not that great.

Magda: Gets me around – that's all I want really. Where would you go?

Jahandar: Don't know, France maybe – Paris. I'd like to go to Paris.

Magda: That would be a long drive. You'd have to learn some French.

Jahandar: I'm good at languages – see how quick I learned English.

Magda: Yes, very impressive. There are probably lots of things I don't know that you are good at Jahandar. I'd like to drive to the north of Scotland. That's a lot of miles but it's beautiful up there.

Jahandar: I once went on a long drive with my Dad and uncle, but that was before . . . [*After a significant silence*]

Magda: I think it must be difficult when thoughts about your family come into your head. It's OK with me if you want or need to talk about them. Whenever.

Jahandar: [*Remains quietly looking out of the window*].

Comment

Magda uses the drive in the car as an unthreatening and non-confrontational context for communication with Jahandar. Ferguson (2011: 110) refers to the non-face-to-face communication within a car which is 'a site of practice where vitally important opportunities for meaningful communication and therapeutic work with children arise'. The car is also a place where the social worker can get away from the busy demands and distractions of the office.

Acting on advice from her supervisor, Magda reduces pressure on Jahandar and provides space for him to begin to test the water of her responses in relation to his past experiences. Jahandar is now ready to speak when they reach the community centre.

Kohli emphasizes the use of narrative as a means of establishing a sense of pride, self-worth and responsibility which contrasts with negative and punitive narratives that have currency in the host community. A UASC, he states, is seen as 'a burden to the state, an illegal entrant, a criminal, worthless and unwanted refugee which is often what he feels about himself' (Kohli and Mitchell 2007: 69). A social worker can, through enabling the child's narrative to emerge, make the child feel emotionally safe and secure. Weld (2009) promotes effective rapport in communication, where the child feels a sense of security from knowing that there is a competent reliable adult who can be trusted to support and protect them.

> *At the community centre, Magda has brought large sheets of paper, felt pens and stickers. They eat their food and she uses this time to maintain the friendly, casual momentum from the car journey to engage Jahandar and continue rapport building about food, football, and travel in cars.*
>
> *When they finish eating . . .*

Magda: After our last conversation at Monica's I thought it might be a good idea for us to work together to help me understand how you are feeling and what we can do to make things a little better. If you're able to tell me how you would like things to be we could try and put a plan together; a plan for you that you have helped to make. What do you think?

Jahandar: What do you mean a plan, who said I need a plan?

Magda: Well, you did say you didn't want to live at Monica's anymore and even though you were very upset when you said that, I think it's important to check that it is the right placement for you. Things change, don't they? Maybe you're ready for a change.

Jahandar: [*Silent but nods his head*]

Magda: It's not just about where you live. Perhaps there are other things we can do.

Jahandar: Like what?

Magda: OK, why don't we sit at those tables where we can write and even draw our plan if we want to?

Jahandar: I don't want to write anything.

Magda: That's OK, I can write, and you can tell me what to write. I can be, like your secretary, and you can draw. I'm no good at drawing, can't even make a straight line.

Jahandar: I'm not drawing pictures, that's kids stuff, no way. [*He is smiling however*]

Magda: What I have in mind is not really about pictures but some diagram or spaces that might help us to work things out; shapes or images that mean something to you and can hold your ideas, your feelings, important people, things like that. Sometimes it makes the talking easier.

Magda then asks Jahandar to draw the diagrams, one for the past, one for the present and one for the future. She explains that he can also write about problems and worries, good things, hopes and wishes. He uses different colours as he chooses to represent people, places, objects and the feelings associated with them.

Jahandar draws a tandoor oven to represent the past, a football for the present and a computer for the future.

Magda: OK, that's excellent. Where would you like to begin?
Jahandar: [*Thoughtful if a little unsure*] Don't know. Suppose the football, that's for NOW – that's easiest.
Magda: Good idea. You can include people, places, things you like doing and anything you want.

In very small writing, Jahandar tentatively and neatly writes football, Arsenal, English, Kabul T-shirt, friends – Afzal and Khalid, The Koran, mosque, kabab, sticky rice. He writes social worker, laughs and crosses it out. Magda is encouraging him throughout and the list generates some conversation about cooking and food that Jahandar misses from home. He also includes movies and refers to a movie he went to with his auntie when he was little and on holiday in Kabul. Jahandar then puts the pen down and sits back in his chair as though withdrawing. Magda waits a few minutes.

Comment

Jahandar refers to his Kabul T-shirt, an object from which he is rarely separated. This is his only remaining tangible connection to his past. Kohli and Mitchell provide context for the importance of such transitional objects to UASCs: 'Our world is ours and we experience ourselves as ordinary people enduring the rough and tumble of our lives without being blown away, because many pegs hold us in place, whether they are people, owned spaces, belongings or documents that confirm our entitlement to remain and be proper within our territories.' For child migrants 'the pegs are uprooted, places abandoned and people and possessions lost in the process of departure from home towards another place, often unknown . . . a transition from a complex and detailed life to one full of risk (Kohli and Mitchell 2007: xiv).

Magda: How about I write some good things about you, in a different colour?
Jahandar: [*Nods his assent*]

Magda writes 'Good student, hard working, intelligent and kind'. She gives examples as she writes and refers to feedback she has received from teachers and Monica. Jahandar, re-engaged, includes Monica in the football. when it appears as though he has finished, Magda encourages him to move to one of the other pictures. He hovers over the oven picture then writes 'Afghanistan'. After a long silence he writes 'night time, 2008'. Magda reminds him that he can include anything – feelings, people, etc. But Jahandar appears to have finished and moves to the computer picture. Magda then writes his name with its meaning around the top of the football: 'Jahandar – owner of the world'. He is suprised and very pleased by this.

Magda: That's really good Jahandar, and when you are ready you might want to add more to the tandoor picture. This will help with your plan.

Jahandar: I have nightmares and I think I shout in my sleep. That's what Sam says.

He writes down 'horrible dreams' in the picture of the football.

Magda: Monica hasn't said anything to me but maybe she hasn't heard you shouting. I know we don't know a lot about your past Jahandar, but we do know it can't have been easy leaving your country and your family, and the little you have said about the journey was frightening and lonely. Maybe there are more things you can put in this tandoor.

Jahandar: [*Shakes his head*]

Magda: Don't worry, that's OK. I am hoping that you will be able to talk about it sometime, maybe a little more when we meet next week. You've worked hard today. Is there anything you want to put in the computer picture before we finish up? All this will really help me to say the important things at your review.

Jahandar writes the following in the third picture: good grades, uni, live with friends in Melrose Avenue, learn better English, get more money.

Jahandar: Can we finish now?

Magda: Yes sure – shall I keep the drawing for you – or maybe you might want to keep it to add to it?

Jahandar: Yes OK – I will keep it.

Magda drives Jahandar back to the foster carer's and arranges a time with him for the following week. At the next meeting Jahandar reinforces his wish to live at a residential children's home in Melrose Avenue where he knows some friends from Afghanistan. He does not dislike the foster placement but it is difficult for him being in a family environment as this is a constant reminder of his loss and separation from his own family.

Comment

Magda will present a report to the resources panel which is set up to ensure that appropriate placements and other children's resources are provided. She will need to use the power derived from her knowledge of Jahandar's situation, his wishes and best interests in order to influence the panel and achieve the resources for the placement at Melrose Avenue. The relationship Magda has so carefully established with Jahandar brings to life the importance of *power with* him enabling her to support him in planning the future of his choice.

The panel will be keenly aware that a foster placement costs much less than placement in a children's home. Jahandar's life story will provide some rationale for a change of placement in spite of the financial implications and, with this in mind, Magda's report includes, with Jahandar's agreement, the drawing which clearly demonstrates his wishes.

The panel will be chaired by a senior children's services manager and will include the service manager, a placements manager and professionals from health and education services. If the panel reject Magda's recommendation she will be faced with a situation of conflict.

Thomas and Killman (2002) defined five possible responses to conflict. Each response leads to different probable outcomes. It is important to consider what the consequences might be for Jahandar's future given Magda's possible responses and her positive use of *power with* and *power to* in representing his interests. The following are some responses that Magda might make for you to consider:

Competing: assertive and unco-operative. In this response Magda is determined to defend a position which she is convinced is correct. She will use whatever power is appropriate to achieve her end in attempting to win the argument. The cause is more important than the sustaining of the relationship with the panel members.

Magda: I can't believe that you haven't listened. All that work that we did that was so difficult and painful for Jahandar – what was the point? Your decision will place Jahandar at risk and he will self-harm again I'm quite sure. The budget can't be everything – what about this boy's future and safety? What am I supposed to say to him now?

Accommodating: unassertive and co-operative. Magda yields to the other's point of view and obeys orders, even if she prefers not to, and her own concerns become neglected. It is seen to be better to ignore the differences rather than to be in open conflict and undermine managerial relationships.

Magda: I know all about the budget. It's a real shame for Jahandar though and I don't know how he will cope with your decision but I will try and help him understand. I will explain how the council has cut the funding for children's services. I'm sure he will be reasonable even if disappointed.

Compromising: moderately assertive and co-operative. Magda attempts to seek some middle ground and to find a mutually acceptable solution. Some concessions may be gained or a temporary solution reached. There is the perspective that a common view can be reached if people on both sides give and take.

Magda: I will see if Jahandar is willing to reconsider his view but also you could see if money might become available next month. I'd be grateful if you would take this to the Director and explore other options.

Collaborating: assertive and co-operative. Magda attempts to reach agreement through identifying the problematic areas and trying to seek creative solutions to them. Conflict is seen to be the result of tension and to be resolvable.

Magda: I'd like to meet with the resource manager this week and see if we can think of some other way forward. Jahandar will take this decision quite badly – I didn't raise his hopes but he really needed some good news as he has been through so much. I'm sure we could find another solution if we looked hard enough. Of course his safety must be paramount.

Avoiding: unassertive and unco-operative. In this response Magda does not pursue her own concerns or those of the panel. The issue may be postponed or sidestepped as she feels helpless and unable to change things for the better.

Magda: I give up. I've done everything I can on this for Jahandar. It's not my fault there isn't any money. I think it's time for me to get some new cases – this work just gets so depressing at times like this when there's just nothing else I can do to help him. Can you give him your decision in writing?

Communication: theory

Ethnocentrism

If the social worker in this case study does not inform herself fully about what is known and also likely to remain unknown about Jahandar's experiences, she will not be able to respond to his needs in a culturally sensitive way. However well meaning, caring and dedicated she may be, without this knowledge she will probably unwittingly act in an oppressive way based on the power of her cultural position. 'It takes little imagination to recognise that communication between members of cultures perceived to be in a hierarchy of dominance are likely to be influenced by the power dynamics involved' (Thompson 2011: 33). Magda would be likely to act ethnocentrically by assuming a similarity of culture given her own experience as a migrant of loss and separation. It is important that she does not impose her own stereotypes in her work with Jahandar. She may not know what aspects of his experience she was discounting because of relying on her own view of the world. Culture is a very powerful factor in communication, as it is a means by which we make sense of our day-to-day interactions. It shapes thinking and behaviour and reinforces the social order.

Thompson defines ethnocentrism as meaning 'reasonably taking your own culture as your starting place in the world but then taking the not-so-reasonable step of assuming that one's own culture is the only true way and that other cultures are inferior' (Thompson 2011: 194). Those who exercise power in a dialogue tend to interrupt, control who speaks when and control the topic under discussion. They also define and control use of names and titles and reinforce social distance between themselves and the young person. In the first dialogue, Magda has her own preoccupations and has some impatience in pursuing her own agenda rather than reaching out to enable and facilitate Jahandar's narrative and as a result he becomes defensive and uncommunicative. Intercultural communication must also be situated in a political context and grounded in an understanding of human rights and social justice. In Jahandar's situation Magda needs to gain an understanding about oppressive immigration policies and legislation and to consider how she can use her power as a professional to promote his rights. Kohli and Mitchell refer to the social worker's experience of having little power to make substantial change in the service provision for young people and mirroring the young person's sense of powerlessness (2007: 69).

Habitus

Bordieu's concept of habitus provides an informative theoretical context for the social worker. Habitus is a relationship of meaning between people. When any two people communicate there will be one with a sense of power over the other derived from their status and position in society. This leads to a set of unspoken rules about who can speak when, whether they will be heard and whether their points will be defined as of value. Habitus is acquired through practice as we learn how to function socially making reference to deeply ingrained patterns of behaviour, feeling and thought. Thompson referred to these being like wallpaper as we forget they are there and take them for granted as they seem to have little bearing on our conscious decisions. When we confront an unfamiliar cultural situation we may become anxious and unsure: 'when we enter into communications with others we are likely to be influenced by the many taken for granted assumptions that form the habitus' (2011: 25). Depending on their social status and power in the social hierarchy, some will have greater cultural resources of influence and therefore are more able to exercise power. This is also referred to as *cultural capital*. Some, through greater advantage in education and upbringing, will be in a stronger position to influence others and to communicate with them. Someone with less *cultural capital* will find it difficult to be heard and find voice.

Power is, of course, embedded in processes and structures as well as in personal interaction and when Magda faces the resources panel which has, in part, been set up to gatekeep resources and contain budgets, she has to identify how she can maximize her professional power in order to represent Jahandar's needs considering his diminished *cultural capital*. If Magda finds voice at the panel then Jahandar will have found voice via his social worker. Social workers can deploy their power to assist or obstruct the struggles of the oppressed ((Lymbery and Butler 2004: 49). Seen in this context Magda bears a very weighty responsibility which has its roots in the quality of her interaction with the young person but extends to her perception of the discriminatory politics of immigration and breaches of children's rights.

Communication: methods

Phatic communication

Phatic communication is smalltalk designed to place the other person at ease, break the ice and build rapport. It is based around neutral topics such as the weather and 'is very significant in terms of forming or sustaining relationships . . . and lubricates the wheels of social interaction' (Thompson 2011: 90). The feedback from phatic communication, such as how someone responds to a simple greeting, is important as it will signify how further communication may develop. Sometimes communication about difficult topics is sandwiched inbetween phatic communication, making it more bearable. Once rapport is built and safe topics are defined, the young person can dip in and out of these safety zones while they speak about distressing subjects. In the third dialogue, Magda speaks with Jahandar about football which she knows is a safe topic. This would have probably relaxed him into conversation if she had not then made a comment about his quietness which placed him on the defensive. Later in the same dialogue she does engage him in talking about driving and this leads to him being able to begin to speak about his painful experiences.

Responding to silence and non-verbal communication

Thompson outlines the various bodily movements which accompany speech and add meaning to it (2011: 102–103). This may be through facial expression, eye contact, certain postures and fine motor movements such as fidgeting, trembling, twisting hair or biting nails. How close a social worker is to someone, and whether they turn towards them or away, is significant, as are the messages of authority conveyed through formal or informal clothing and professional 'props' such as diaries and mobile phones. Some aspects of non-verbal behaviour may indicate cultural or religious identity and good practice demands that social workers, unsure of the meaning of behaviour, seek clarification rather than making assumptions and following stereotypes.

At the start of dialogue one, Magda does not recognize non-verbal messages in Jahandar's awkward silence as he shifts about on the sofa and pulls at his jumper sleeves. He presents a nervous smile clearly conveying a message that he is not sufficiently comfortable to talk about the incident of self-harm. He asks Magda if he can get a drink. She agrees but immediately refers back to her need for information – once again not recognizing the pressure he is being put under to discuss very painful experiences. His escape mechanism in suggesting a drink should have been understood and respected, and as it was of his own choosing may have led to him feeling more relaxed and empowered to find voice. When she persists further he becomes startled and his heightened state of anxiety creates a communication barrier and he begins to blame himself for the self-harm. Any attempt to plan together is now foiled. Thompson refers to the concept of *emotional holding*, a term used to refer to the process of helping the child to feel emotionally safe and secure (2011: 62). It involves forming a rapport to the point where a child gains a sense of security from knowing that there is an adult who can be trusted to support and protect them. A child will not feel *held* without good communication, but a 'held' child will be much easier to communicate with than one who does not feel secure.

Kohli describes young people who, when interviewed at point of entry into the UK, remain silent about their lives or are economical with the truth. They commonly present as compliant, polite yet troubled children who are anxious about speaking to strangers and have often been told by their families to reveal nothing about their lives. The child will fear adding any detail which might adversely affect their claim for asylum. They also worry about their families being traced and placed at risk if their whereabouts are revealed (Kohli 2006).

Silence is also of course a response to trauma and deep disturbance. It is a means of surviving loss and separation from everything and everyone they have known, and provides a barrier to the feelings of pain. Silence can be healing and allow the child to cope with everyday life in a new country. This is a concept Kohli refers to as *psychological hypothermia* which has a protective function as slowly the child can *thaw out* and proceed with their life. Social workers need to understand the dynamics of this silence and how to support the child in moving from a superficial, limited and contained *thin* account which is constructed for the receiving authorities as a path to citizenship, to a *thick* account which has emotional content and allows distressing detail to be safely and confidently communicated. Progressing to a *thick* account takes place following acknowledgement and acceptance of the silence and mystery surrounding the child who states the *thin* story they have rehearsed and been told to tell. The *thick* account is multi-layered and complex. Once told, and shared with a trusted person, the experiences can be integrated and deep-seated emotions and memories explored slowly over time. Always, the social worker must progress at the pace of the child and be sensitive to their cues when they demonstrate by their behaviour, verbally or non-verbally, that they can say no more and then, through speaking and telling, the child will be enabled to reconstruct their life and move forward. The therapeutic dimension to the communicative relationship between a social worker and a child can never be underestimated.

Recognizing and responding to non-verbal behaviour is important in addressing power imbalances. When working with young people the social worker will always be in a position of power through status, size, age and other relevant factors such as gender and ethnicity. Children will tend to agree with adults in order to please them – this is known as the *omniscient adult effect*. Techniques can be used by the social worker to reduce the social distance between themselves and the child such as not towering over them but communicating with them at their level, sitting alongside or playing on the floor and through wearing less formal clothes. Care must be taken to be authentic in these efforts as children will immediately note the insincerity of a social worker who speaks poor *street language* or pretends to understand aspects of youth culture which they are not familiar with. When Magda speaks with Jahandar in the car, she is reducing the social distance between them and he becomes more relaxed in her company. The quality of the child's account increases when there is less social distance as there is less likelihood of the child feeling intimidated and seeking to please or feeling anxious and withholding information.

Storytelling is an example of a sensitive method of communication for children who come from cultures with oral traditions and are familiar with stories being used in teaching. It is promoted by Dr Melzak from the organization Medical Foundation for the Care of Victims of Torture who states: 'We are trying to give them coping strategies . . . but instead of saying directly what they saw or did, we deal with it through displacement. They can be extracted through stories which create safe arenas to talk. The therapy helps *to put the child back together*. One of the coping strategies if you are traumatised is you stop using your imagination.' The stories can be used to recall and develop strategies to deal with problems and build resilience for a child cut off from the usual support networks (Chamberlain 2007).

Advocacy

In representing Jahandar's views to her managers, Magda needs to advocate for him. The advocacy role may be described as linking people with resources or acting as an intermediary. The advocate supports or speaks on behalf of the service user emphasizing their rights to services. Boylan and Dalrymple discuss the pressure that social workers experience from managers responsible for allocation of scarce resources and how they need to be willing and able to challenge authority in order to represent the young person's needs and best interests. They comment that critical practitioners as advocates need to 'appreciate the power of the dominant discourse and need to understand how concepts of power, oppression and inequality determine personal and structural relations' (2009: 46). Of course, in addition to the social worker's advocacy an independent advocate can be recommended.

Containing and bearing witness

In the third dialogue, Magda achieves a gentle breakthrough with Jahandar using her capacity to work at his pace and be guided by both his ambivalence and his tentative emotional engagement. Kohli and Mather comment that being a witness is being still, unafraid, honest, kind and emotionally robust: 'it is harder than rescuing but ultimately more productive because it lets refugees name and exorcise their own demons and ghosts in the process of self recovery'. They advise that social workers develop the skills 'to stay still long enough to bear the pain of listening to the stories of great loss as they emerge at a pace manageable for the refugee' (2003: 206–208).

Kohli clarifies that unless young people themselves chose to disclose they should not be pushed to give an account as they themselves may have witnessed death, torture and sexual assault and also may have been forced participants. They may also feel guilty about surviving when others close to them have died or remain in danger: 'They seem to have the strengths of much older children and yet the vulnerability of much younger children so that the chronological and developmental ages may well be at variance. They live with the paradox that someone they love has sent them away and will remain anxious about the safety of those why stayed behind' (2006: 206).

Communication: ethics and values

Meaningful connection with the child's experience

Social workers need to learn from research studies which have ascertained the views of UASCs. This knowledge will assist them in communicating and reaching out into the world of the young person. While each UASC's experience will be individual, there are some commonalities, and with increased understanding the social worker is more likely to have confidence in being an effective advocate. Obtaining the child's views is essential if social workers are to feel more empowered to promote their interests and to challenge those who use authoritarian systems to oppress the interests of those without UK citizenship.

The young UASCs interviewed for various research studies have emphasized their need for safety. They said they wanted caring adults to keep them safe, who understood the complexity of their experience and connected them to networks that were meaningful to them for support. This includes access to specialist legal representation, the health service, social services, immigration and police (Williamson 1998).

A strong sense of isolation added to their level of fear and anxiety: 'I feel isolated because I am from a different culture and a different country' (Children's Society 2008). Blackwell and Melzak (2000) found that young people wanted a sense of belonging to an adult, school or social group and to be able to think about the past in a safe context. They wanted choices to integrate culturally but also to mourn aspects of their culture which have become inaccessible such as access to home food and cultural affiliations. One young person said: 'I have access to resources I couldn't have at home but it has been a bad thing to be away from my family' (Children's Society 2008). It was important not to rush to replace the search for meaning in a young person's culture. To assist them in moving forward, they needed careers advice and education. They wanted to learn about the British way of life and to have social activity.

ECPAT (2011) campaigns for the appointment of legal guardians for unaccompanied children in order to advise them of their human rights and connect them to relevant organizations.

The right to an interpreter

A report by Refugee and Migrant Justice emphasized the importance of proper use of interpreters in work with UASCs to counter poor practice, as demonstrated by young people's accounts below:

> *The interpreter was from Iran and I am from Afghanistan. I told the interpreter that I did not understand him properly . . . I felt powerless and*

frustrated. Even the identity card that was given to me by the Home Office said that I was a Pashtu speaker but I speak Dari. I didn't know what any of the questions were about and I thought I was going to be taken to prison . . . I felt that no one understood me.

When I arrived in the UK I was in a bad state. I felt very weak and I had a bad headache. I went with another person to hand myself in to the authorities. I just wanted to be safe. It was strange when I was interviewed. They used a telephone. I have never used a telephone before and I don't think I was listening properly and I couldn't understand the interpreter.

(RMJ 2010: 8–9)

An interpreter provides language support and transmits an oral message from one person to another across the language barrier. A translator is a person who provides language support, who transmits a written message from one person to another across the language barrier. An interpreter is not an advocate for the child or a source of cultural advice.

Magda has been working with Jahandar for some time and knows that he speaks good English even though Pashtu is his first language. Jahandar has a right to an interpreter which must be respected if he is not to experience disadvantage because English is not his first language. Particularly when discussing difficult and emotional issues, Magda should have offered him the opportunity to have an interpreter in case he wished to express complex feelings in his first language.

Interpreters are specialist professionals and need to be involved in planning the interview and deciding whether the young person would need them to 'stand by' in case they were needed. Interpretation may be simultaneous as the social worker and young people speak or consecutive with each person waiting until the interpretation is complete. For the young person to feel included throughout, the social worker must address them directly, using the first person, making eye contact and not speaking at the interpreter. The social worker should sit in a triangle positioning themselves facing the child with the interpreter to the side. The social worker needs to keep sentences short and be constantly aware of the interpreter's signals. At no time should the social worker leave the interpreter alone with the young person as this might expose the interpreter to difficult situations and be unsafe for either party.

It is important for the interpreter to be briefed about possible content so that they can prepare and also raise with the social worker any difficulties such as words and concepts which are not easily translated in another language. Some interpreters may not be willing to use particular words such as those with sexual connotations and this needs to be clarified prior to the interview to allow time to seek an alternative interpreter. Strategies for addressing any difficult situations should be discussed and agreed and the interpreters should be asked to check for any misunderstandings. Checks should be made with the young person that the interpreter is not known to them or the family so as to maintain confidentiality, and the young person should also have a choice as to the gender of the interpreter. The interpreters may feel distressed after the interview and time for debrief is important.

Communication: the knowledge base

Facts about UASCs from Afghanistan

The UK is a primary destination for young people from Afghanistan, especially for the Pushtun which is the majority ethnic group in the country. The UK has a well-established community of Pushtun and there is a perception of good educational and welfare services within a diverse society (Mougne 2010: 30). In 2010, of the 1717 unaccompanied children seeking asylum, almost a third of the applications were made by young men from Afghanistan (this was a reduction from 50 per cent in 2009). UASC applications from Afghanistan have continued to decrease although the reason for this is not understood (Home Office 2011).

About one in ten UASCs are denied asylum and approximately 75 per cent gain only discretionary leave to remain until the age of seventeen and a half (Kohli 2011: 316). UASCs are mainly between the ages of 16 and 17. About 6 per cent of all looked after children are unaccompanied young people mostly in London and the South East. Across the country there were, in 2010, about 4200 UASCs being looked after by local authorities (Sirriyeh 2011). There are reports of serious mental health problems among those who are living independently and have exhausted their rights to appeal. They are threatened with deportation and the idea of return to Afghanistan represents a personal failure and betrayal of trust (Mougne 2010: 31).

An unaccompanied child whose asylum is refused should only be returned to his or her country of origin if there are adequate reception arrangements available in that country. Sending children back to a conflict zone could not possibly be in their best interests and therefore all Afghan children in the UK are in need of international protection from armed conflict. However, social workers need to be aware that there has been widely condemned government pressure to deport UASCs back to Afghanistan and therefore it is likely that young people will have fears of being deported (Travis 2011).

In February 2011, the UN Committee on the Rights of the Child reported critically on children's rights in Afghanistan. The Committee expressed concern over the deaths of hundreds of children as a result of attacks and airstrikes by insurgent groups, international military forces and the Afghan national army, stating that armed forces responsible for the killing of children had not been held accountable and that the grievances of families had not been addressed (UN Committee 2011: 29).

Legal and policy context

The legal and policy context relating to UASCs is complex and highly contested by organizations representing the interests of children. Social workers, in order to advocate effectively, need to have a comprehensive and critical understanding of the statutory constraints relating to this work and be well versed in current government documentation and guidance as well as the reports from children's rights groups and campaigns. This is a specialist area of social work with a specific knowledge base which has relevance to social workers in all areas of practice.

Asylum is protection given by a country to someone who is fleeing persecution in their own country. It is given under the 1951 United Nations Convention Relating to the Status of Refugees. To be recognized as a refugee means that after leaving the country of origin the young person has a well-founded fear of persecution in that country for reasons of race, religion, nationality, membership of a particular social group or political opinion.

Following an application for asylum, a child, while their application is processed, is usually given discretionary leave to remain in the UK for a determined period of time after which they have to apply for an extension. A referral is made by UKBA to the local authority who have a duty to accommodate the child under Section 20 (Children Act 1989) because the child has no one with parental responsibility to care for them. If there is doubt about the age of the child, UKBA will request an age assessment by the local authority. If the asylum application is initially refused, the young person has a right to appeal to the Asylum and Immigration Tribunal.

The paramountcy of the child's best interests applies to all children including asylum seeking, refugee and migrant children irrespective of their nationality, immigration status or statelessness. This principle is enshrined in the European Convention on Human Rights (Council of Europe 1950), The Human Rights Act 1998 and the Children Acts 1989 and 2004. The UNCRC (Articles 19 and 37) and European Convention (Article 3) state the rights of children to be protected from torture, inhuman or degrading treatment or punishment and from all forms of abuse.

The child's immigration status should not affect the quality of care, support and services that are provided as a result of the assessment and if children are refused asylum status then agencies must also work together in making sure that the children are equipped for their future life on return to their countries of origin. The guidance states that social workers must build close links with the UKBA case officer responsible for resolving the child's immigration status sharing relevant information about age assessments, medical and social needs and efforts made to trace family members. Any concerns relating to the child's need for protection from harm must be investigated in line with the local child protection procedures in the area where they are living in the same way as for any other child.

Section 55 of the Borders, Citizenship and Immigration Act 2009 places a duty on the Secretary of State to make arrangements for ensuring that immigration, asylum, nationality and customs functions are discharged having regard to the need to safeguard and promote the welfare of children in the UK. While it is the UKBA, an agency of the Home Office, that has duties to maintain a secure border, and to ensure controlled and fair migration policy implementation, it is statutory guidance (Home Office 2009: 2.4) that UKBA staff must adhere to a code of practice defining their legal duty to ensure *good treatment and good interactions* with children. They must make timely referrals to agencies providing ongoing care to children and identify and refer children who may be at risk of harm to the statutory agencies (Home Office 2009: 2.22). The code of practice states that children's best interests are a *primary* although not necessarily the only consideration.

Migrant children are excluded from the remit of the Department for Education as the Home Office takes the lead on policy which results in a two-tier system as they are seen as immigrants first rather than children and do not receive the protection they need (RCC 2011). As one example, many UASCs enter the UK without valid documentation and may be prosecuted if they are over the age of criminal responsibility (10 years). Children's rights groups recommend that in this situation children should have an absolute defence in law (CRAE 2011).

Accommodation: Section 20 (Children Act 1989)

The presumption is that children with no parent or guardian to turn to in this country would need to be looked after under Section 20 including during the time while an assessment is conducted. Since R (Behre) v Hillingdon (2003) (known as *the Hillingdon judgement*), the duty of local authorities to provide aftercare services under provisions of the Children (Leaving Care) Act 2000 has applied also to former unaccompanied asylum seeking children until they attain the age of 21 or beyond if in full-time education.

Bhabha and Finch (2006) concluded that vulnerable children, particularly those over 16 years, were being placed in unsupervised accommodation inadequately supported by the local authority. Government funding to authorities had been reduced and they noted reluctance to use Section 20 partly because of the cost of resourcing their leaving care duty.

Brownlees and Finch (2010) identified a severe shortage of foster carers for UASCs. Yet practitioners said that foster care was generally the best placement option as children gained more intensive support, felt safe, were more likely to succeed educationally and gain help in seeking contact with family members. Foster care was also more suitable in relation to language, culture and religion. The young people felt included and did not feel pressured to speak about painful experiences (Sirryeh 2010). However, and particularly relevant to Jahandar's case, the experience of being suddenly in the midst of a different family may be overpowering for some young people and they may feel conflicting loyalties between the foster carers and their own family. Sometimes they may feel guilt about their living conditions in comparison to those of the family left behind. Fostering does not necessarily provide access to a peer group where the young people can share similar experiences, whereas in a children's home there may be other children from a similar background (Hek 2007: 111–113).

It is important to recognize that fostering is itself a culturally defined concept which may be unfamiliar and in some cultures might be suggestive of slavery and domestic servitude. 'It is most important to consider the views and wishes of young refugees themselves, rather than have a *blanket* approach or strict agency position', as some children, for example, prefer foster placements so that they can learn the language quickly (Hek 2007: 114).

Entry into the UK: the journey

The journey can cost thousands of pounds and parents sell houses, land and possessions to raise the money. Some children's journeys are paid for in segments by their families and the children have to wait at each stage, at the mercy of the agents, until payment is made. Most children are reported to have had no idea what the journey would entail or how long it might take – from six months to years. The most common route from Afghanistan is via Iran to Turkey, Greece, Italy and then to France, UK and the Netherlands. Some go via Austria and Germany and on to Scandinavia and others avoid Greece and go via the Balkans. Boys have reported travel from Iran being in trucks or buses in cramped and difficult conditions sometimes for weeks, travelling in small boats between Turkey and Greece and some have witnessed others drowning in rough sea crossings. The agents are described as controlling the young people through fear and intimidation and beatings are commonly reported (Mougne 2010: 16–21).

Entry into the UK: the arrival

The campaign organization Refugee and Migrant Justice (RMJ 2009) found that children were frequently interviewed on arrival without a legal representative or responsible adult present. The children felt constantly disbelieved and reported their health and other basic needs as unmet. The young people's accounts of arrival speak for themselves:

> When I was first arriving in lorry, lorry went in airport . . . me and other boys were found by police. The police arrested me, I was taken to police station and fingerprints and all that. I was scared.
>
> (Children's Society 2008)

> I was detained for a long time. I was moved from one place to another and asked lots of questions by different people . . . I was disorientated and confused. I didn't know what was happening. I was afraid that I was going to be sent back to Afghanistan to be killed . . . The person who interviewed me was angry with me. They asked me how I got to England and warned they could send me back.
>
> (RMJ 2010: 14)

Detention of unaccompanied children at the ports of entry

The damaging impact on children of being detained is well documented (Lorek et al. 2009; Burdett 2010). The Refugee Children's Consortium stated that 'the detention of young people has a detrimental effect on their mental and physical health. Its effects include weight loss, sleeplessness, bed-wetting, nightmares, skin complaints and severe mental health difficulties including self harm, depression and symptoms of Post Traumatic Stress Disorder' (RCC 2011).

Research by the Children's Society (2011a, 2011b) found that between May and August 2011 697 children were held at Greater London and South East ports of whom a third were UASCs. There was little information from the Home Office about this form of child detention, about why children were being held, their age or for how long. The Prisons Inspectorate published three reports about children kept in short-term holding facilities (HMIP 2011). The inspectors reported a terminal with 'no dedicated child-friendly interview rooms and children interviewed in stark rooms with chairs attached to the floor'. Sometimes there was no telephone available and children were held on average between 8 and 12 hours with some for longer periods of time up to 30 hours.

Age disputes

Although UKBA staff are required to accept the local authority age assessment, unless there is countervailing evidence, about 28 per cent of children claiming asylum, about 1200 children, have their age challenged by the UKBA every year.

The Refugee Children's Consortium and their member organizations have supported 'numerous clients who have been made destitute, detained or accommodated as adults but later identified as children' (RCC 2011). Where a child is incorrectly assessed as an adult, or older than they actually are, this has profound effects on the child including being detained with adults, being housed with adults, missing out on education, not having the protective support of a corporate parent, and a loss of identity leading to self-harm and depression. In addition the young person loses the safeguards provided to unaccompanied children.

CASE STUDY AND REFLECTION

Zubeir's experiences as an unaccompanied asylum seeking child

Jahandar's experiences in local authority care provide a window into his unmet needs. This account by Zubeir, a young person in similar circumstances, requires us to appreciate how complex the use of power is and how important it is for social workers to use it effectively. Zubeir (anonymized) was aged 16 when he arrived in Dover. Zubeir's problems began when American and British forces invaded Afghanistan. His house collapsed when neighbouring buildings were hit in an allied bombardment. As a result of the blast, Zubeir sustained serious injuries to his legs. This has caused permanent damage, and UK consultants have said he requires an amputation. He remains in a great deal of pain. Zubeir's baby brother and younger sister were killed in this incident and his mother was also injured.

"I was 16 years old when I first arrived into the UK. When the Americans and the British invaded Afghanistan our village was bombed. I was about nine years old at the time. I was badly injured by the blast.

There were bad people in our village. Some years after the bombing my father was killed . . . My father's family started to abuse and threaten me and the rest of my family. My mother's family arranged for me to be taken to a safe country. My uncle told me that the British would protect me because they believe in human rights. My uncle arranged my escape and instructed the agent. I had to do everything that the agent said. My family told me that I had to because they were taking me to a safe place.

The escape and journey was frightening and painful but all I could do was hope and pray to God that I would be safe. At times I was in agony. The agents beat me and the other boys a lot. We were passed from one agent to another like animals. The pain in my leg would be so bad that I would faint and fall unconscious. Because of my injuries I was too slow and could not move at the speed they wanted, so they would beat me. They used to hit me with belts and sticks.

We travelled through lots of countries but I didn't know which ones. We also went through a country called Greece. I remember that we were in France and I had to live in a place called the 'jungle'. Lots of people lived there, adults and children. It was horrible. We lived outside and it was cold. Sometimes we had nothing to eat. Good people from a church used to give us food there. But sometimes the food was not enough.

The agents were very abusive and would hit me and the other children. I was also attacked by a group of men when I was living there. They stabbed me in the back. This was three or four days before I arrived into the UK. Thankfully I didn't die but later my stab wound became infected and blood and pus was coming out of it. I felt so alone and threatened. It was terrifying there. I was surrounded by older men and had nobody to support me. I was very ill.

We could not have a wash or a shower. I had not had a shower for about one and a half months. I had a rash all over my body. I kept itching and itching but then I started to get big lumps on my body that also had pus in them. My thighs were the worst but I couldn't stop scratching them. I think that they were abscesses.

The agent finally forced me to hide in a refrigerated lorry. It was very cold and it made me feel very ill. I was in the lorry with adults and another young person. We were forced to stay on top of some boxes. The boxes had yellow stuff in them. It could have been yoghurt or butter, I can't be sure. We got into the lorry during the evening, and the UK officials found us not long before sunrise the next day. It was so cramped and I was so cold. I was also in a lot of pain from my old leg wounds, the stab wounds and the abscesses.

When I arrived in the UK, I was in such a bad way. The UK officials put some stairs on the lorry so that we could get out. When we got off the lorry we were put into cars. It was hard to walk but no one said anything to me. We were then driven to a place in Dover; I am not sure what the place was. I did not understand what was happening and no one told us. All of us were then taken into a big room. We had to sit in chairs and wait for a long time. I was searched and had to take all my clothes off. I was in my pants for some time because the UK officials were searching my clothes. It took a while before they returned my clothes.

Then each of us were interviewed. I waited from the early morning until the afternoon before I was interviewed. I think it was in the early afternoon but I cannot be sure exactly. I waited a long time and I was in a lot of pain but I had to do what the UK officials said. I was very frightened and I didn't know what would happen to me.

I remember that someone came in and gave us something small to eat, which was in plastic. We were not asked if we needed to see a doctor or if we were well. I did not know that a doctor could come there. No one asked me about my health. I just sat in the chair . . . They kept asking me questions about why I came here, my journey and what happened in Afghanistan . . . After the interview I was told to wait for some hours.

I was then taken to a hotel and after a couple of days a lady came to see me and I think she was from social services. She took me to the doctor straight away because I was very ill. I have been in the care of social services ever since. My asylum claim was later refused because the UKBA said that I did not offer enough information during the interview that took place when I first arrived. But because I am a young person I was given special leave to remain. My social workers have helped me so much since I came here. They look after me and care for me. They are like my family. If I need anything I can call them. Sometimes I think I am being a burden on them so try not to call all the time. I do not know where I would be if I did not have them to call.

Since being in the UK I have found out that one of my brothers has been killed by the bad people in Afghanistan. I would be dead now if I was not here. Sometimes I think I should be dead. My key worker and social worker have tried their best to find me help and support for my problems. Sometimes I have panic attacks and I get scared easily. I have to take a lot of pills that the doctor has given me and they make me very drowsy but I still can't sleep. My key worker explains to me that it is important that I take these pills.

I have also made some friends here in the UK and they help me too. They don't always let me sleep over at their house because I scream in my sleep. My neighbours also complained about my screaming but I don't know I am doing it. I just hurt so much. The pain in my body and heart is too much for me sometimes. I have started to hurt myself to get rid of the other pains that I have but my key worker talks to me a lot and tells me I can't do this.

I recovered from the stab wounds, but my doctor here says that my leg wound is so bad I need an operation. I don't know where I would be without the support I have from my friends and social services. I feel blessed and I feel protected by those around me. But the government here does not want me. I am scared that they want to return me to Afghanistan. I am scared that if I return I will be killed like my brother. When I look on the TV I see that British soldiers and government ministers are being killed in Afghanistan and they have all this protection around them. How would I protect myself? I can barely walk for more than 15 minutes without pain."

This account is from the publication 'Safe at Last? Children on the Front Line of UK Border Control (RMJ 2010: 4–5). Similar and other accounts may be found on the following website: http://www.freedomfromtorture.org/search/node

Questions to aid reflection

Drawing on the knowledge presented in this chapter and your learning from analysis of the script consider the following questions:

 What key knowledge about children arriving in the UK from Afghanistan would have enabled Magda, in the first dialogue, to have responded more sensitively to Jahandar's needs?

 How does the application of the theory of Habitus help to keep Jahandar's wishes as the focus of their communication?

 Consider the positive and appropriate use of silence in painful and complex communication with children?

 How does Magda prepare for potential conflict in her role as advocate for Jahandar?

 How does Magda use power with *to connect with Jahandar and promote his best interests?*

 How does Magda use power to *in presenting her report to the Resources Panel?*

Agencies and websites

Social workers need to be informed about the key agencies involved in this area of work so that they know where to access specialist advice and support.

Children and Families Across Borders (CFAB) (International Social Services). CFAB's mission seeks to promote and protect the rights of these families, children and other vulnerable adults across international borders, according to the UN Convention on Human Rights and on the Rights of the Child. www.cfab.uk.net

Children's Rights Officers and Advocates (CROA). A network of children's rights workers contributing young people's views to policy and practice. www.croa.org.uk

Immigration Law Practitioner's Association (ILPA). Professional association of lawyers and academics practising in immigration, asylum and nationality law. www.ilpa.org.uk

Medical Foundation for the Care of Victims of Torture. Provides rehabilitation, counselling and therapy. www.freedomfromtorture.org

National Coalition of Anti-Deportation Campaigns (NCADC). Supports community-led campaigns for justice in the asylum and immigration system, with a focus on supporting people facing forced removal. www.ncadc.org.uk

Refugee Children's Consortium (RCC). This is a group of NGOs working collaboratively to ensure that the rights and needs of refugee children are promoted, respected and met in accordance with the relevant domestic, regional and international standards. www.refugeechildrensconsortium.org.uk

Refugee Children's Rights Project. Access to advice and legal representation for children and empowering professionals to be effective advocates for children in line with the UNCRC. www.childrenslegalcentre.com/index.php?page=refugee_childrens_rights_project

Refugee Council. Advice to asylum seekers and refugees, supporting other organizations' refugee work and promoting the rights of asylum seekers and refugees. http://www.refugeecouncil.org.uk

Recommended reading

Crawley, H. (2012) *Working with Children and Young People Subject to Immigration Control: Guidelines for Best Practice*, 2nd edn. London: Immigration Law Practitioners' Association.
Kohli, R. (2006) The sound of silence: listening to what unaccompanied asylum seeking children say and do not say, *British Journal of Social Work*, 36: 707–721.
Kohli, R. and Mitchell, F. (eds) (2007) *Working with Unaccompanied Asylum Seeking Children: Issues for Policy and Practice*. Basingstoke: Palgrave Macmillan.
Matthews, A. (2011) *Landing in Kent: The Experience of Unaccompanied Children Arriving in the UK*. London: Office of the Children's Commissioner.
Thorpe, A. (2011) The use of power in social work practice, in T. Okitikpi (ed.) *Social Control and the Use of Power in Social Work with Children and Families*. Lyme Regis: Russell House.

5 Persistence: Overcoming organizational barriers in family work with a disabled child

Introduction

Chapter content

There is no doubt that if children are to gain protection, and services when in need, the voices of those professionals close to the world of the child must be heard. There have been numbers of situations where social workers have *blown the whistle* on poor practice and abuse of children. For example, in the London Borough of Islington in the 1990s social workers raised concerns about children being sexually abused in children's homes and their evidence led to 13 inquiries and much media and political response (Fairweather 1998; Harris and Bright 2003; Davies 2006). More recently, Nevres Kemal, a social worker in the London Borough of Haringey, sounded the alarm about child protection procedures prior to the death of Peter Connolly (Fairweather 2008c) and on the Channel Island of Jersey, Simon Bellwood disclosed abuse of young people within the custodial systems (Ahmed 2007).

If social workers are unheard, vulnerable children will also be unheard. This chapter explores the role of the social worker in raising concerns from the earliest stage when they observe or witness poor practice. Organizations need to be responsive at this stage so that concerns do not escalate and children gain their right to services. This chapter provides examples of the complex communication skills which enable persistence in raising concerns effectively.

The ethical and practice requirements of social workers are explicit in a range of codes, legislation and guidance, yet achieving justice and human rights for service users is an increasingly difficult task in the context of extensive welfare cuts and the deregulation and privatization of children's services. Calder (2008) outlines the risks of organizational dangerousness when an agency is not listening to staff and does not create a safe working environment where concerns are well received, explored and addressed. An open, learning culture in the workplace supported by non-defensive management and embedded in policy and protocols will ultimately be supportive of the rights of vulnerable children and families.

This chapter examines the need of a social worker to challenge a manager's approach to the protection of a disabled child. The context of the manager's response is one of reduced resources and the consequent pressure to raise the threshold in *child protection* cases by defining them as *child in need*. The social worker needs to persist in communication with his manager in his determination to provide the appropriate service to the child and family. In doing this he also communicates effectively with his colleagues both within and outside his agency. The chapter also considers how the social worker might have persisted in raising his concerns if his manager had not listened. It concludes with a recent serious case review concerning the death of a disabled child which provides an example of how the authorities did not recognize the child's need for child protection strategies.

Summary of the script

In the first dialogue, the school nurse raises her concerns about the health of a child, Manisha, in her school. The social worker, Aseem, raises this professional concern with his manager in the second dialogue, suggesting a child protection response as appropriate. His manager disagrees and insists on keeping the case at the threshold of *child in need*. In the third dialogue, Aseem speaks with the parents and sees Manisha and her sister Tara and his concerns increase. In the fourth dialogue, school staff emphasize further concerns to the social worker, but in dialogue five the manager remains resistant to a child protection approach and the social worker remains unheard. Through persistence, the social worker engages the multi-agency network and his team colleagues in exerting pressure on the manager. The sixth (alternative) dialogue demonstrates the manager's listening response to the social worker's concerns and that of the team. If the manager had not responded positively, the social worker would have needed to think carefully about the next steps he could take in striving to protect the child. He would need to consider how to comply with his duty of care as required by his contract of employment and as defined in the professional standards (HCPC 2012c).

The script: through persistence, a social worker, Aseem, with the support of the multi-agency network and through challenging managerial resistance, ensures the application of child protection procedures for, Manisha, a disabled child

Setting the scene

Manisha is a British Asian girl aged six who lives with her parents and older sister Tara. She has pauciarticular juvenile rheumatoid arthritis and is identified as a *disabled* child and a *child in need* (Children Act 1989). Children's services are involved due to concerns regarding Manisha's increasing levels of pain and refusal on the part of her parents to consider conventional medical intervention, which they fear has detrimental side effects. They insist on alternative remedies and take Manisha regularly to a homeopath. The most pressing concern is that, without medication, Manisha may lose her sight. Her symptoms sometimes go into remission and at these times she goes to a ballet class which she loves.

First dialogue

Children's social worker, Aseem, receives a call from the school nurse

School nurse: Hi Aseem, I'm phoning with an update and further concerns regarding Manisha Desai.

Aseem: Hello. I'm glad you called. It was on my list to phone you today for a catch-up.

School nurse: Well, it's not good I'm afraid. Like I indicated at the last network meeting Manisha is really struggling with her mobility and is often in pain. It's very concerning, distressing even, to see a child in such discomfort. Other children are finding it difficult too, the class teacher has said, and there appears to be no shift in the parents' attitude to the conventional treatment route. I'm not convinced they understand the dangers.

Aseem: Yes, I appreciate it is very difficult, and the school staff have been really supportive. I will take it back to my manager again but there is a strong view here that Mr and Mrs Desai know what they are doing and that they are entitled to explore the alternative/complementary therapy route. I'm not saying I absolutely agree with it mind.

School nurse: Well as far as I'm concerned I have a duty to Manisha's health and well-being and I find it unacceptable that a child has to experience ongoing pain and discomfort in order to satisfy the parent's right to explore the options, however well they articulate their case.

Aseem: Yes, the GP has explained clearly the paediatrician's most recent report advocating for medication and the implications of delay.

School nurse: More and more I am thinking that this case should be within child protection procedures. Surely the possibility of a child's eyesight deteriorating is risk enough – a threshold of significant harm?

Aseem: It would seem so – but at the same time, it's not as though the parents are disengaged or difficult and it would be hard to prove that they don't have their child's interest at heart. The principle of working in partnership can be a very persuasive argument for not escalating the case.

Comment

Aseem is rightly concerned at possible over-identification with the child's parents/carers. There is a risk of identifying indicators of abuse as attributable to the stress and difficulties of bringing up a disabled child and overlooking Manisha's needs.

School nurse: Well I think it is unacceptable and in all this discussion we are in danger of overlooking what is actually happening to Manisha. Can you go back to your manager and discuss it again? I will record that I have requested child protection procedures and the reasons given, and I will speak to the rest of the school staff who know the child. They think similarly to me I'm sure.

Aseem: Yes, please do and I will speak with my manager before the end of the day. It would be helpful if you could send me a report of your most recent concerns. It might help to convince people on this side. I think we are coming from the same position.

School nurse: OK will do. Thanks Aseem.

Comment

Maintaining the centrality of the child's best interests is the critical focus for this case. Aseem begins to collate evidence from other professionals who know Manisha well. This enables him to evidence a persuasive case to his manager when he needs to persist in his efforts to protect Manisha from harm.

The important role of the school nurse in monitoring, tracking and integrating information from a variety of sources was emphasized in a study of three serious case reviews concerning disabled children (DfES 2006).

Second dialogue

Following his conversation with the school nurse, Aseem speaks with the team manager about his increasing level of concern about Manisha.

Manager: Hi Aseem. Yes, we need to have a quick discussion about the Desai case. I know you spoke to the school nurse this morning and I've just had the safeguarding nurse on the phone. She is really pushing for a child protection conference. Honestly, they'll only be satisfied if every case is child protection.

Aseem: They do have a point in this case I believe, and it is a health issue after all.

Manager: That may well be but we have knowledgeable parents here, co-operative mostly and they love their child. If we push this into child protection procedures we are likely to lose that co-operation and I expect they will be very intractable.

Aseem: But there is the issue of potential loss of sight without the methotrexate medication and . . .

Manager: Yes, yes, I am aware of that but there was some uncertainty about timescales in relation to her sight, and the parents are very worried about the side effects of the medication.

Aseem: I was going to add that there is also the issue of the pain Manisha experiences and the impact of this across the board – her emotional well-being, education, socialization, etc. Apparently she is becoming more and more isolated in class because the other children find it difficult to be around her – her unhappiness.

Manager: I wonder if that might be a little over-dramatic. The thing is, *we* have to decide on thresholds and at the last count child protection cases in the team are nearly 40 per cent up on what they were a few months ago. It is not sustainable with current resources and our last vacancy is not going to be filled.

Aseem: But surely we can't let those issues determine our threshold otherwise children will fall through the gap and then what? I think it is very difficult to defend that position.

Manager: It is not that simple unfortunately, and where there is a chance that a case can be held as a child in need – which is where I want this one to remain – we have to take a strategic position. Look, I know you are very worried for this child but let's keep our heads here. I can't imagine that Manisha's parents don't know what they are doing – they are educated people, architects I think, and they probably have good reasons to be suspicious of western medical intervention with its emphasis on medication. The family have a right to their cultural perspectives on health treatments. Do another visit to the family and encourage them to comply. Health need to see we are taking them seriously – whatever we think.

Aseem: Of course – but I'm not confident it will progress things. I'm also not happy with the assumption that it is a cultural issue. From my understanding, traditional alternative treatments can be complimentary to western medical interventions.

Comment

Aseem makes an important challenge to the manager's assumption. Without evidence she has linked the parental choice of treatment to their culture. Aseem rightly raises this as a form of professional dangerousness which risks losing focus on the child.

Third dialogue

Aseem makes a prearranged visit to the family home at a time when Manisha is home from school so that she is included. Mr and Mrs Desai prefer to speak with Aseem on his own first. Manisha and her sister Tara, aged 12, are in a nearby room. Aseem observes a comfortable child-centred home.

Aseem: Mr and Mrs Desai, thanks for agreeing to the visit. I'm here because the school nurse has ongoing concerns for Manisha.

Mrs Desai: Well that's understandable. She doesn't agree with our way of managing Manisha's condition. So it's neither new nor surprising.

Aseem: That may be but she is very concerned about the degree of pain Manisha is experiencing in school and the impact on her mobility.

Mr Desai: But we have been through all this and it is becoming tedious to have to continue explaining ourselves, and indeed having to defend *our* choices for *our* child. Our homeopath has assured us that the treatment regime he has prescribed is effective and has proven results. We are satisfied with that. Are you aware of the different remedies and how they work separately and in combination to improve Manisha's mobility with the least amount of pain?

Aseem: But that's the problem as I understand it from the school nurse – the pain is not improving, and the consultant is quite clear about the additional risk to Manisha's sight. It seems the homeopathy does not address that very serious issue, serious risk in fact.

Comment

Aseem maintains his focus on Manisha's experience rather than being distracted by the parent's view of treatment.

Mrs Desai: Look, we know you have to do your job, and we appreciate your concern, but there must be more needy people than us who require your attention. We are not unaware of the problems for our child and we are quite capable of ensuring her safety. Do you seriously think we want her to be in pain?

Aseem: I believe you want the best for Manisha but there appears to be a reluctance to consider some of the risks that we discussed at the last meeting. Have you taken up the paediatrician's offer of a second opinion?

Mr Desai: This is ridiculous. We don't believe it is necessary to have another opinion. Our lives are busy enough and we anticipate the same old response – a cocktail of toxic tablets for a six-year-old, supporting no one but some pharmaceutical multinational. Are you aware of the side effects of the medication that has been prescribed for Manisha? No, I didn't think so, well that's what we consider dangerous for our child.

Comment

Aseem is now struggling in his response to the parents because he is insufficiently informed about the side effects of the medication recommended by the consultant. He feels overwhelmed by the parents' arguments and is anxious to see Manisha on her own.

> *This conversation is interrupted when Tara runs into the room. She is angry and upset with Manisha and refers to her as a baby and useless. She says it's no wonder Manisha has no friends. Mrs Desai attempts to calm the situation, while Aseem observes Manisha in the adjoining room looking very tearful and dejected. Mrs Desai takes Tara from the room and suggests it is not the best time for Aseem to speak with Manisha as had been previously agreed.*

Aseem: It must be quite a strain generally having a child with a disability in the family.

Mr Desai: We're used to it. This is the real strain, having social workers involved!

Aseem: There are supports we can provide – maybe Tara could do with some as well.

Mr Desai: Tara is fine. She just gets frustrated with her sister and can get quite nasty but we're on top of it.

Aseem: How do you mean?

Mr Desai: Unfortunately, she likes to pinch Manisha, but rest assured we are dealing with it.

> *Mrs Desai returns to the room.*

Mrs Desai: Sorry about that – we just need to keep them apart for a bit till they both calm down. The thing is Aseem – we love our children and are completely committed to them. Although we really don't want to be involved with social workers and find it very stressful, we have attended all appointments, allowed all your visits and we have listened to all the views from different professionals. But, at the end of the day we are Manisha's parents and we have a right to a family life and to provide for our children as best we see fit. We wouldn't dream of putting either of our girls at risk. For goodness sake, I've even given up my job for them. We also know much more about the treatment regime advised by our homeopath and, with respect, if you don't have that knowledge you are not in any position to be offering advice about alternatives.

Comment

Although the Children Act 1989 emphasized the child's right to a family life and for professionals to work in partnership with families, the paramountcy of the child's best interests takes precedence over all other principles in the Act.

Aseem: I understand all those points but I have a responsibility to Manisha and central to my concern is the level of ongoing pain she experiences and the opinion of the medical experts who are very worried that Manisha may lose her sight if she does not take the medication. It is my duty to take this very seriously. In addition she is unhappy and isolated in school and her performance is significantly affected. I would like to come back and see Manisha and speak with Tara too if that's OK. We do want to support you as a family and make sure that Manisha is not unnecessarily suffering. Should we make a time now?

Mr Desai: Best to phone us. I'll see you out. By the way, I'll send you the website where you can get up to speed about the side effects of the drugs they are prescribing for Manisha.

Aseem returns to the office and shares the outcome of the home visit with his manager. He was particularly unhappy that he had not succeeded in spending any time with Manisha alone. He reinforces his earlier points regarding parental intransigence about the medication, lack of apparent insight into professional concerns, and possible blocking of his contact with Manisha. He also identifies a new concern regarding Manisha's relationship with her sister. Aseem suggests a strategy meeting identifying neglect as the risk. The manager continues to challenge Aseem's analysis. She identifies the stress of being parents of a disabled child impacting on the family dynamic. She once again draws on cultural differences in regard to treatment options, rejecting Aseem's suggestion for a strategy meeting and reminding him of the benefits of using a strengths-based supportive approach. She reiterates the need to keep down the numbers of children subject to protection plans.

Fourth dialogue

Aseem receives a further call from Manisha's school. The designated child protection teacher questions the lack of a child protection response to the school nurse's referral and raises an additional concern.

Teacher: I don't understand why this case is not being taken more seriously. All of us who work with Manisha at the school are extremely concerned. We really shouldn't have to plead with children's services to get action on a case.

Aseem: Please be assured I am taking your report and concerns very seriously – it is just taking a lot of persuasion and persistence here to take the case to the next level. I also want this case in child protection procedures as the parents are failing to see past their own concerns about the medication. They are very stuck and I worry that they are beginning to withdraw.

Teacher: Well, Manisha presented with bruises on both arms today and wouldn't say how they happened. Something is not right here. If this were a child from a poor family I wonder if the response would be different?

Aseem: Perhaps, but a more urgent concern I believe is the current child protection statistics and the lowering of thresholds due to recent high profile serious case reviews. My manager is very resistant. I expect she is under pressure too.

Teacher: As far as we are concerned in school we're not referring to a statistic but a child and it is beginning to feel dangerous. Are you aware that recent appointments with the hydrotherapist and the physiotherapist have also been missed because both therapists said they couldn't bear to see Manisha in so much pain and that she had not been given pain relief.

Aseem: No, that's a new development and definitely worrying. I wasn't informed. Look, leave it with me and I will speak with my manager again. The bruises are possibly from the sister's pinching, which parents told me about this week.

Teacher: The parents have been advised by the head teacher to take Manisha to the GP, which they said they would do.

Aseem: I will push again for a strategy meeting. Manisha should probably be seen by a child protection doctor. I will get reports from the hydrotherapist and physiotherapist.

Comment

In addition to addressing concerns about neglect of Manisha's needs in relation to medication, there is now a possibility that she is suffering physical
harm as there are unexplained bruises. Aseem needs to be persistent in taking
forward the voice of the child as identified by those close to her in the education and health agencies.

Fifth dialogue

*Aseem approaches his manager once again in an attempt to have the concerns
taken more seriously and to push for a strategy meeting*

Aseem: I have just received new information about Manisha Desai from
the designated child protection teacher. She presented in school today
with bruises and recent appointments with her hydrotherapist and the
physiotherapist have been missed. They are very concerned in school at the
increased level of pain too and the lack of attention to the future loss of her
sight if her parents continue to refuse Manisha methotrexate mediation.

Manager: Is any of this actually new information Aseem? If I remember from our
last conversation, the Desais were open and honest about the pinching and
said they were dealing with it.

Aseem: The missed appointments are new and the level of concern being generated at the school is really high. They feel very strongly that we are not taking
this seriously enough.

Manager: On the contrary, I have spent more time this week discussing this case
with you than any other individual case in the team.

Aseem: I think that's because I am very concerned too. I agree with the school
staff though.

Manager: We have to be careful about overreacting in these situations. We children's services make the decision about thresholds, not the school.

Aseem: Is it not a multi-agency responsibility at a strategy meeting?

Manager: This is important Aseem. The decision to call a strategy meeting is
the responsibility of the team manager. But, let's get back to the facts of
the case. This is a family who are co-operating and with the exception of
a couple of recent missed appointments they have not resisted our
involvement. I believe there is opportunity for further persuasion to engage
with conventional medical treatment.

Aseem: If we had a strategy meeting and all the professionals sat around a table
to discuss it, perhaps the focus on Manisha would be less diluted.

Manager: You are not listening to me Aseem. There will not be a strategy
meeting for this child and that is final.

Aseem speaks with the GP who is satisfied with the family's explanation that a friend in school caused the bruising and that they are dealing with it appropriately. Aseem's concerns now escalate because different accounts are being given by the parents for the bruising. He is worried that more information may be hidden. The team manager, however, remains sceptical and suggests that the parents may be getting confused given the pressure from professionals. Aseem is also anxious about the reaction of the school when he feeds back that he has been unable to gain management agreement to a strategy meeting.

As he predicts, school staff are shocked and angry and, with the support of the head teacher, they threaten to involve the chair of the Local Safeguarding Children Board (LSCB). Aseem immediately emails this development to the team manager, who is not available to speak with him. Later the team manager comes to Aseem's desk and is furious and dismissive. 'So be it – my decision stands' is her final comment. Aseem makes a record of the exchange on Manisha's file.

However, following representation from the chair of the LSCB, and the intervention of the local authority child protection manager, a strategy meeting is convened the following morning.

Information is shared, debated and analysed and a plan to progress the enquiry is formulated. Manisha is to be interviewed and a child protection conference convened to consider risk of harm.

Manisha is interviewed by a police officer and social worker in a child interview suite, in compliance with the Achieving Best Evidence (ABE) guidance (Ministry of Justice 2011). After some rapport, she spoke about her ballet classes and how much she enjoys dressing up, wearing her ballet shoes and watching the ballet on television. More recently the pain in her legs has been so bad that she has missed classes and is falling behind the other pupils and this has made her very sad and lonely. She loves her parents but doesn't understand why they can't make the pain go away. She is also unhappy because Tara pinches her.

Alternative dialogue

The sixth dialogue represents an alternative approach to achieving a more satisfactory outcome at organizational level and demonstrates a less confrontational managerial response to Aseem's persistence. When reading the following dialogue consider:

- How can Aseem persist in challenging his manager about his concerns?
- What support does he need to take the issues forward with management?
- What expertise can he draw on to further inform his view?

- How will Aseem communicate with his manager to influence her perspective?
- What knowledge base will assist Aseem in his discussion with his team manager?

Sixth dialogue

At a team meeting Aseem raises the difficulty he has experienced in getting protection for Manisha. He describes being caught between pressure from other agencies, the hostility towards him from the family and his own determination not to lose the focus on Manisha. His views reflect the general atmosphere and concerns within the team. Various social workers contribute their experience of being blocked by the manager from moving child in need cases into child protection following their assessments. In his next supervision, Aseem draws on these team experiences and the culture of dissatisfaction.

Team manager: OK, great! That's all your cases discussed. Did you have anything else on your agenda.

Aseem: Actually, yes. I want to discuss some outstanding issues with regard to the Manisha Desai case.

Team manager: Oh! Has something new come up, what's the problem?

Aseem: It's nothing like that. Things are progressing fairly well for Manisha as we discussed earlier. I want to raise the difficulty I experienced in getting this case into child protection.

Team manager: Oh Aseem! Do we really need to go back there – is there anything to be learned?

Aseem: Well yes, I think there is. And, other team members have expressed similar concerns about progressing cases, particularly when the risk is not so clearly evidenced and establishing the threshold is based on professional judgement. The Munro report puts significant emphasis on the importance of professional judgement and we need to be implementing the findings (Munro 2011).

Team manager: As a social worker your responsibility lies very clearly with the family, the children in the family. It isn't as straightforward when you are a manager. I have a more diffuse duty of care. While I am also responsible for safe practice and outcomes, part of my role is to be accountable for the allocation of resources and ensuring we meet targets, performance indicators, standards, etc. Sometimes very difficult calls have to be made and I don't expect everyone to agree with me. Most of the time I try and protect staff from having to engage in these discussions in order not to distract them.

Aseem: But most of us in the team are aware of those pressures and when we push against resource-based decisions that don't account for our assessments, particularly around risk, it is because we are scared that something more dangerous may happen. Realistically, we are worried about children and ourselves in that context.

Team manager: Yes, I do appreciate that the disagreements are not personal and I also appreciate that most of the team are very committed to the families they work with. Thinking more broadly than the Desai case, we also have to ensure that we don't become too risk averse as unnecessary intervention at a statutory level can be disastrous for a family.

Aseem: But it is also very problematic for families when cases drift with unacceptably high levels of concern, and the deterioration can be almost imperceptibly slow yet critical in relation to safety for children.

Team manager: Yes I can see that. These are the cases that we need to have robust discussions about. I'll have to think about how to address these concerns Aseem, and come back to the team.

Aseem: We did come up with some ideas in the group that might be worth considering.

Team manager: Great – give me the headlines now as we don't have much time and if you could put them in an email I can give them my full attention later. I can also bring them to the senior management meeting next week.

Aseem: First, as thresholds can present such difficulty – we thought it would be useful to have a fortnightly slot at team meetings to present a case that someone is struggling with. Space and direction for discussion on complex cases can make what Lord Laming refers to as 'respectful uncertainty', a practice reality that will help with casework as well as with building staff confidence, particularly around articulating concerns and translating them into degree or level of risk (Laming 2003).

Second, we would also like to invite someone from the LSCB to a team meeting to discuss the impact of budget cuts and resourcing on our direct work with families. That might help to share the burden and ownership of the problems we are dealing with.

Third, more targeted training would also help – particularly with our multi-agency colleagues, focusing on how to address conflicts in our assessments.

Fourth, ways of managing stress arose for discussion, so we want to look at staff support in relation to that too, particularly in relation to our workloads.

Finally, these are the issues and concerns that as a team we need to have acknowledged and addressed. We believe that if our concerns are validated, with some follow-through from management, we will have more confidence in our work with service users.

Team manager: Thanks Aseem. I know it is not easy to raise issues such as these, and having thought them through in this substantial way adds credibility to the concerns. I do appreciate your honesty and your professionalism. I recognize too that I have a duty of care to you and your team colleagues so I will give these points my serious consideration, and we will have a full discussion at the next team meeting to find a way forward.

Comment

Aseem's persistence in pursuing his important ethical and practice issues towards a relatively successful resolution is underscored by the following:

- He has prepared carefully, consulting with and gaining the views of his team and multi-agency colleagues.
- He has utilized the expertise of the local child protection manager.
- He has identified possible solutions to the problems identified, drawing on the recommendations of current policy documentation.
- He has presented his views in an assertive, professional manner without recourse to over-confrontation or aggression.
- He has continually restated the basis of his view, as located in the rights of the child and his professional accountability.

If Aseem's manager had not listened he would have had other options for taking matters forward. First, he would need to try and raise the issues through mechanisms internal to the agency via senior management. He could also speak with the chair of the Local Safeguarding Children Board which has a duty to seek to resolve conflict between agencies in safeguarding children in the locality. If he were a member of the British Association of Social Workers he would be entitled to representation and advice. If he were a member of a trade union such as Unison or Aspect he would have been able to invite a union official to meet the team and discuss how the union might act to represent their interests with senior management. If all internal mechanisms had been exhausted then he could, as a citizen, see his own Member of Parliament and discuss the difficulties with him or her. As an employee of the council, however, he is not allowed to contact a local councillor or speak with the media as this would be a disciplinary matter without manager's agreement.

Whistleblowing is defined as 'the disclosure by an individual to the public or to those in authority, of mismanagement, corruption, illegality, or some other form of wrong-doing in the workplace' (HCPC 2012b). Social workers need first to raise concerns through the internal mechanisms. They need to clarify and gather evidence, raise the concerns with managers individually and collectively with colleagues, set out the evidence in writing, raise the matters through other internal means such as supervision, team meetings, grievance procedures and consultation processes. Any difference of view between a social worker and team manager must be recorded on the service user file and in the supervision notes for future reference. Managers will need to decide whether the reported situation is actually or potentially unsafe and set their views in writing, outlining whatever steps they will take to rectify a situation.

Only if all internal mechanisms are exhausted and without resolution, a social worker may access the agency whistleblowing procedures. These protocols will provide information about how to raise a concern and details of the individual within the organization who is the appropriate contact point. At every stage the social worker must keep accurate records.

Social workers are within the remit of the Public Interest Disclosure Act 1998 which provides protection from victimization and dismissal for workers who speak out against corruption and malpractice at work. Statutory protection requires the making of a *protected disclosure* in good faith and not for personal gain. Social workers need to consider the importance of compliance with professional codes and that this may mean challenging their employer. The charity Public Concern at Work provides advice to whistleblowers in confidence (www.pcaw.org.uk) and the trade union Aspect has published a useful guide about staff duties and rights with a set of pro-forma letters to assist staff in raising issues correctly (Kline 2010). If all internal mechanisms have been implemented without resolution then the concerns may be escalated externally. This would usually be to a *prescribed regulator* such as Ofsted or the HCPC. Useful advice with regard to raising concerns and whistleblowing is to be found on the HCPC website (2012a, 2012b).

Multi-agency work is another way of supporting effective social work practice. Guidance such as *Working Together to Safeguard Children* (DfE 2010) requires shared decision-making through statutory multi-agency fora such as strategy meetings and child protection conferences. Decisions made in these meetings, as outlined in Chapter 2 and 3, enable shared responsibility in the most complex of cases and support individual actions to protect children. Any dissent to such decisions is formally recorded and explained.

Communication: theory

Social model of disability

I have no legs
But I still have feelings,
I cannot see
But I think all the time,
Although I'm deaf,
I still want to communicate,
Why do people see me as useless, thoughtless, talkless,

When I am as capable as any,
For thoughts about our world.
                    Coralie Severs, 14 yrs (Unicef 2008: 2)

The social model of disability is a way of understanding the position of disabled adults and children and the world in which they live emphasizing a rights perspective. It is a challenge to the medical model which focuses on changing disabled people through medical intervention rather than changing the disabling barriers in society. Kennedy and Wonnacott commented that 'the terminology "disabled children" is quite different from the phrase "children with disabilities". The former describes the social model where there are disabling barriers and the child is "dis-abled" by society whereas the latter uses the word "disability" to describe the child's impairment . . . and ignores the political dimension of prejudice and discrimination which should be acknowledged and addressed when undertaking any assessment' (2003: 175).

Kennedy and Wonnacott expressed concern about the *children first* principle (Children Act 1989) which helped practitioners to focus on the disabled child's needs as a child: 'now the pendulum has swung too far and practitioners are not focussing enough on the child's identity as a disabled child and all that it means to live in a discriminatory world' (2003: 185). This approach has reinforced a tendency to deny the child's disability. It is clear that the effects of oppression may be as devastating to the child as the effects of the impairment itself – often even more so.

The social model enables examination of the differential structures providing services to disabled children and the impact this may have on service provision. Murray and Osborne (2009: 15) emphasized the importance of 'ensuring clarity of responsibility within children's social care for safeguarding disabled children between specialist disabled children teams and family social work referral and assessment teams'.

There is a risk that general teams may lack emphasis and knowledge about the child's disability, and disability teams may lack child protection expertise. In Manisha's case the team manager located in a children's team fails to link the complex details of the child's disability with parental capacity to protect. An Ofsted report (2012) which involved a survey of 12 council child protection services and analysis of 173 cases identified that the lack of rigour in the management of child in need work increased the likelihood of child protection concerns not being identified early enough. When disabled children did become subject to child protection plans, there was a marked improvement in their outcomes, effective action was taken to reduce the risk to them and in the majority of cases they made good progress.

Cooke found that social workers working in a specialist disability team may find difficulty separating their *supportive* role from their *investigative* role if a family is well known to them (2000). Kennedy and Wonnacott comment that being assessed for *parenting capacity* might seem offensive to a family requiring services and support (2003: 187). Joint training in both child protection and disability equality issues is essential across all staff in both teams with also the availability of specialist safeguarding disabled children advice (Murray and Osborne 2009: 19). Ofsted found that a significant number of authorities had no such specialist training (2012).

The social model equally allows analysis of how disabled children may experience bullying. 'One of the biggest barriers faced by disabled children is that they are commonly seen as their impairment. Their age, gender, ethnicity, religion and culture that make up their unique individuality are subsumed into this one dimensional labelling' (NSPCC 2003: 58).

Negative attitudes towards disability cause disabled children to be more vulnerable to bullying and abuse by peers, and the internalization of oppression can result in compliant victims who may see themselves as deserving of harmful or neglectful treatment as between Tara and Manisha in the script. This can lead to 'an incidious and relentless pressure that can dominate their lives leaving them feeling depressed and withdrawn. Adults may see the disabled child's behaviour as a part of their impairment rather than identifying bullying as a reason for the change' (Murray and Osborne 2009: 21). The Office of the Children's Commissioner found that disabled children can be twice as likely as their peers to be targets of bullying behaviour (OCC 2006) and research evidence shows 'the devastating impact that this can have on their lives' (Mepham 2010: 19). Children with visible disabilities may be particularly likely to meet with patronizing, hostile or demeaning comments which can have long-term emotional impact. A Unicef report recommended the message of *ability*: 'Having a disability is not a bad thing. It can even be something to be proud of. We are all different and all have different abilities . . . This book calls on all people from all nations to honour and respect us just the way we are' (Unicef 2008: 5). The Disability Discrimination Act 2005 places a duty on schools to demonstrate how they are promoting disability equality and local authorities are required to be proactive in eliminating disability related harassment and in promoting more positive attitudes towards disabled children (Mepham 2010: 27).

Communication: methods

Touch

Kitson and Clawson (2007: 176) draw attention to how disabled children are handled routinely by different carers and medical practitioners which makes them more vulnerable to abuse. The use of touch by a social worker, as an aspect of communication, is always a matter for professional judgement.

Ferguson refers to *professional touch* such as handholding while walking or through playfully picking up a toddler to say hello. He argues that touch is an important part of ethical good practice conveying caring and healing: 'Every worker should be prepared to touch children as a routine part of their practice and do so without question when certain situations require it' (Ferguson 2011: 105). Picking up a baby or young child can be an important way of discovering information about their well-being. However, he urges caution if a child has been sexually abused, for instance, they may interpret touch as abusive. 'Sometimes a touch is right and sometimes it isn't – it's difficult to explain the difference, if it feels wrong it probably is' (Murray and Osborne 2009: 33).

An NSPCC report commented that the costs for children are high when there is a loss of affection in the care of children and emphasized the importance of a children's rights approach to standards and expectations of staff. 'We know that touch is important to emotional development and we can consult with children about what forms of physical comfort they prefer' (2003: 63).

Personal negative responses to a disabled child may lead to avoidance. Lasswell's theory of communication and perceptual screens (see Chapter 3, this volume) develops the transmission theory concept of *noise* as being the barrier to effective communication. He suggests that a more complex process of communication is relevant as he describes communication going beyond a data exchange and including perceptual screens which are conditioned not only by immediate, situational factors, but also by culture, self-esteem, personality, moods and organizational context (1948).

Personal perceptions of what it means to be disabled affect the social worker's response. Attitudes as well as emotional and physical responses must be explored and understood to counteract barriers to communication likely to cause avoidance and disregard. Uninterrogated feelings can subject a disabled child to the raw disgust or discomfort of a professional attempting to apply meaningful and often sophisticated communication methods.

Each person will have different perceptual screens depending on their upbringing and experience. For instance, are some impairments experienced as more emotionally difficult than others? Which aspects of a child's disability are more or less comfortable to be recognized and understood?

Talking Mats

Talking Mats is an augmentative communication tool providing the basis for communication which assists children in expressing their views. Through the use of picture symbols placed on to a mat according to 'happy, don't know or unhappy', Talking Mats can help children reflect on their lives and what may be changed. The method gives the time and space to think about

Happy   **Don't know**   **Unhappy**

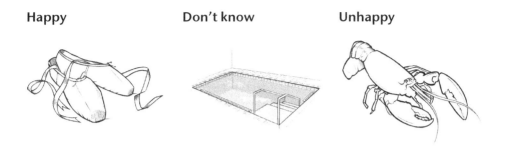

Figure 5.1   Talking Mat

information, work out what it means and say what they feel in a visual way that can be easily recorded. Manisha's mat might have looked like Figure 5.1. Manisha is happy when she wears her ballet shoes. She is unhappy when she is pinched by Tara. She is unsure of her feelings at the hydrotherapy pool as sometimes she enjoys the therapy but often it is very painful for her (www. talkingmats.com).

Achieving Best Evidence in Criminal Proceedings: Guidance on Vulnerable or Intimidated Witnesses including Children (Ministry of Justice 2011)

The guidance for interviewing disabled children as witnesses in criminal proceedings is detailed and comprehensive and states that 'there is rarely any reason why disabled children should not take part in a video-recorded interview provided the interview is tailored to the particular needs and circumstances of the child' (Ministry of Justice 2011: 172). Research has also demonstrated that disabled children are able to provide accurate and reliable evidence in response to open questions that differ little in quality or completeness from that of non-disabled children (Davies and Westcott 1999: 17). The guidance considers preparing and planning for interviews with witnesses, decisions about whether or not to conduct an interview, and decisions about whether the interview should be visually recorded or whether a written statement would be more appropriate.

The guidance requires interviewers to be aware of the extensive differences between disabled children in relation to their social, emotional and cognitive development and their communication skills and to respond to specific needs by gaining specialist advice and considering the need for intermediaries to facilitate the interview process. A pre-interview is recommended which allows detailed assessment of the child's requirements. Specifically attention must be paid to creating a safe and accessible environment with use of communication aids such as drawing to facilitate questioning and recognition of the child's need for medication and breaks. The interview will need to be arranged at a time and location convenient for the child even, where necessary, taking the recording equipment to another location such as a hospital. The interview may need to be longer and questioning may need to be more direct with flexibility in relation to timescales and the use of the phased interview approach. The interviewers will need to have a detailed understanding of the child's world (Davies and Townsend 2008; Ministry of Justice 2011: 10–27).

Yet even though disabled children are more likely to have suffered abuse than those non-disabled, evidence from disabled children has rarely been used in court. It was often wrongly assumed that disabled children would not be able to give credible evidence in criminal proceedings and courts sometimes failed to meet the child's needs with insufficient use of visual recording and intermediaries (Murray and Osborne 2009: 55; Stalker et al. 2010: 5). Although research by Aldridge and Wood (1998: 190) illustrated that 50 per cent of police officers had interviewed a disabled child, none had received any training in interviewing children with special needs. They had little understanding of practical considerations such as the need for wheelchair access or an induction loop for those with a hearing disability or of the detailed requirements for an interview such as toys and props. It was reported in one study that: 'It just reinforces the feeling of not being worthy of all the rights and entitlements of a non-disabled child. There is an awareness for most disabled children that they are struggling and that they are different' (Stalker et al. 2010: 20).

The phased interview approach to an Achieving Best Evidence (ABE) interview

Manisha is interviewed by the police officer and social worker according to the Achieving Best Evidence Guidance (Ministry of Justice 2011). She would have met them before the interview and had an opportunity to understand the interview process. This guidance recommends the phased interview approach which supports good practice in obtaining an account from the child that maximizes the obtaining of good evidence. The aim of the interview is to obtain an accurate and truthful account in a way that is fair, is in the child's best interests and is acceptable to the court. There are four phases: introduction and rapport; free narrative; questioning; and closure. These phases may not always follow consecutively and it is important for interviewers to remain flexible and respond to the child's needs. It may be necessary to return to earlier phases of the interview or to proceed quickly to a later stage. The guidance suggests that any divergence from the basic framework should be agreed by the investigating team. It is rare to conduct an ABE interview with a child more than once but when interviewing disabled children a number of interviews may be required in order to work at the child's pace and to be respectful of their needs.

Introduction and rapport phase

If this phase is conducted in a relaxed and child-centred manner it will set the scene for the main part of the interview, helping both the child and the interviewers to feel at ease. The interviewers make sure the child is comfortable and that physical needs are addressed. The professionals and child introduce themselves using both first and second name and then state what they like to be called more informally giving the child permission to be comfortable with the interviewers. Social workers and police describe their role and it can be helpful to explain that their work involves:

- speaking with children who are sometimes happy and sometimes sad
- making sure children are kept safe
- listening very carefully to children
- taking very seriously what children want to say.

Following explanations about the cameras in the room and statement of the day, date, time and place, the rapport phase enables the interviewer the opportunity to build on their knowledge of the child which they will have gathered from the planning meeting and from the pre-interview meeting.

During the rapport phase the interviewers attempt to put both themselves and the child at ease by talking about neutral topics such as the child's hobbies, friends, school, likes and dislikes. The topic must not include any situation connected with the alleged abuse. The interviewers get alongside the child through play, allowing the child space to talk about their world. This is the time for the social distance between the interviewers and the child to be decreased and therefore lists of questions about school or home are to be avoided as the conversation should be two way and as relaxed as possible, enabling the child to feel comfortable and to speak with ease. This will set the scene for a higher standard of evidence from a child who would be less likely to feel intimidated by the adults into providing the response that they think the adult wishes to hear.

If an intermediary is used then the rapport phase will allow familiarization for the child and the interviewer and for checks to be made to ensure good communication. Drawing and toys can be used to assist the process. A disabled child can be supported in communicating about their day-to-day life during this phase to assist the interviewer in placing any abuse allegations in the context of the child's specific disability and circumstances. This will include the interviewer understanding the child's needs for breaks and to reassure the child in feeling confident to make requests for assistance.

The rapport phase should always be included. If the child wishes to progress quickly to the main part of the interview some rapport should be built in or the interview may be the subject of criticism. Rapport forms the foundation of the interview. At a later stage of the interview, when painful subjects are being discussed, the child might return to the rapport stage to draw breath and gain the courage to proceed further with disclosure. The child will be informed that they can let the interviewer know that they do not understand something, they do not know the answer to a question or if they are not sure how to say what happened and that they must not guess if they are unsure. They will also need to make a commitment to telling the truth which can be agreed by everyone in the room.

The free narrative phase

This is the opportunity for the child to tell what happened in their own words uninterrupted by the interviewer. It is a spontaneous account and high in evidential accuracy. The child describes events as they remember them and so it is rarely a chronological account. The interviewer in this phase is mainly listening but may ask specific non-leading questions to clarify aspects of the account. For example, if the child mentions a car the interviewer might ask what colour the car was or who was in the car. This type of question usually begins with How, What, Where, When or Who. 'Why' questions are avoided as they often imply blame.

Open-ended prompts are also useful during this phase – such as 'Tell me more about that' or 'Help me to understand that a bit better'. Acknowledgement is very important throughout; for example, 'It can't have been easy for you to tell me about these things' or 'Thank you for explaining that to me', 'It would now help me to understand . . .' or 'Please go back to what you were saying about when you were in the car'. This phase is a constant flow between acknowledging what the child has communicated and then helping the child to continue their account. Clarification can be sought: 'I don't want to make a mistake and need to check that I've understood you properly.' The interviewer may need to clarify terms or actions such as relating to specific parts of the body and drawing or toys can be helpful to this process. On no account should the child be asked to point to their own bodies or that of the interviewer or intermediary as this would be abusive. Any sensory perceptions noted by the child are likely to provide important evidence about what has happened. If a child explains how something smelt, tasted or felt, then it is likely that they did experience the event that they are communicating about.

Example of part of an interview with Manisha during the free narrative phase

Social worker: Tell me what happens when you can't go to your ballet classes.
Manisha: My legs hurt too much and I have to rest.

Social worker: Is there something that helps you feel better?

Manisha: Mummy gives me a warm bath. I like that. It helps.

Social worker: What else does Mummy do that helps?

Manisha: She gives me a yukky drink made from flowers. It's OK. Tastes like weird bubble gum.

Social worker: What happens after you've had the drink?

Manisha: Then I rest and watch the TV. Unless Tara comes in.

Social worker: What happens if Tara comes in?

Manisha: She pokes me like this. (M picks up the Fluffy Rabbit on the sofa and pokes it with her finger)

Social worker: Oh dear that doesn't sound very nice. Tell me more about Tara.

Manisha: She hates me. She hates me 'cos I can't play with her very well. I'm too slow. She says I'm no good at ballet. She's no good at anything. She doesn't know anything about ballet.

Social worker: Tell me more about what happens when Tara comes in.

Manisha: She pinches me and it hurts. Like this. (M pinches the rabbit again and again) You wouldn't like that would you?

Social worker: I wouldn't like pinches, no I wouldn't.

Manisha: Where's Mummy?

Social worker: Mummy is waiting downstairs.

Manisha: Can she hear what we're saying?

Social worker: No she can't hear you as she is downstairs. We will see her after but first it's important you tell us some more about how you manage at school.

Manisha: Mummy doesn't like me talking about my hurting legs.

Social worker: Tell me what Mummy says.

Manisha: She tells me my legs will soon get better and to think about other things.

Social worker: What helps to make your legs feel a bit better?

Manisha: Joanne makes them better but she can't when they hurt too much. So then I just sit and wait for school to end or I have to go home and Mummy and Daddy come for me.

Questioning phase

During this phase the legal points to prove about the case will need to be covered in detail and questions used to seek to clarify further the child's account, to be clear about whether or not the child is safe and what action may be necessary to protect the child from harm.

Apart from specific non-leading questions there are open questions, closed questions and leading questions. Open questions do not in any way suggest an answer. They usually elicit long, detailed responses and provide accurate information. These may begin with phrases beginning with words such as *tell, explain* or *describe*.

Closed questions allow for a yes or no response from the child and are generally to be avoided. For example, 'Did your legs hurt at the pool?' would be better framed as 'Tell me where you were when your legs were hurting?' which allows for more options in the response.

Leading questions are those that suggest a response and put ideas into the child's mind, for example, 'Your legs hurt at the pool didn't they?' These are also to be avoided but for some disabled children leading questions might be the only way that they can clearly comprehend the question. In planning the interview, the child's specific communication needs will be clarified and will guide the interviewer.

Closure

During this phase the interviewer thanks the child and returns to the rapport phase to ease the tension. They can use the opportunity to ask the child for some feedback about the interview and their views of any barriers to communication. The interviewer makes sure the child is not distressed and confirms arrangements for returning home.

Communication: ethics and values

Childism in relation to disabled children

Two Worlds
Torn between the ears of
Sounds and Silent,
Uncertain, unable to join . . .
Tears flow . . .
Unknowingly both push away,
Rejected, made to feel
Unbelonging . . .
Sara Leslie, 16 yrs (Unicef 2008: 16)

About one in 20 children (3 per cent) are considered disabled and increasing numbers of children with severe medical conditions now survive into adulthood. They are an oppressed group. The oppression is identified through all the ways in which barriers in attitudes, language, culture, organizations and power relations devalue disability and result in segregation and exclusion. Segregation is the separation of one group by a more dominant group. Inclusion requires a holistic approach applied to every aspect of practice such as the accessibility of the building, suitability and provision of resources and access to disability awareness training. Disabled children are not a homogeneous group and are not only the responsibility of specialist practitioners. Each child should also be seen as an individual with an impairment or disability that is part of their identity and not as a tragic case requiring sympathy

There is limited information available about the circumstances of disabled children in the UK or about the prevalence or pattern of disability. It is known that most disabled children have more than one disability, with severely disabled children commonly having physical, sensory and learning disabilities. Very little research has addressed the views of the disabled children themselves. However, Watson et al. (1999) interviewed disabled children and found that disability was a dominant status in which other differences, such as gender and ethnicity, were secondary. The children said they were constantly reminded that they were different from non-disabled peers and compelled to adopt the behaviour, ways of speaking and walking which most closely approximated the ways of non-disabled children (1999: 15). It has been shown that disabled children from minority ethnic groups experience discrimination compounded by institutional racism (Chamba et al. 1999).

Discriminatory attitudes towards disabled children may include beliefs and myths such as that disabled children are more likely to make false allegations about abuse or that disabled children are less damaged by the abuse than non-disabled children: 'We still come across situations where child care professionals do not believe anyone would abuse a disabled child, where the child's pain and distress is not recognized, where abusive practices are seen to be necessary because of the child's impairment' (NSPCC 2003: 10). Communication barriers impede disabled children's ability to report and describe abuse. Therefore, lack of access to independent facilitators or specialist communication systems and technology are forms of childism impacting on a disabled child's right to be protected. Ofsted (2012) research concluded that professionals did not always take into account that disabled children are more likely to suffer abuse or neglect at home and cases were uncovered where issues of neglect had not been picked up by social workers, particularly in cases with a history of adult mental health difficulties or domestic violence. The report concluded that 'in a sizeable minority of cases decisions were taken that no further action was needed by children's social care. These decisions were not appropriate given the extent of the concerns.' Ofsted's chief inspector commented that 'in some cases the focus on support for parents and their children seemed to obscure the child's need for protection' (Lepper 2012).

Equality of provision

Disabled children should be treated with the same degree of professional concern as non-disabled children. Yet the systems designed to protect all children may fail disabled children. Disabled children may require additional resources to meet their communication needs, particularly with regard to time allocation, accessing specialist advice and services, lengthy enquiries and background checks. Themes from serious case reviews indicate an under-reporting of disabled children in the child protection system and a lack of tracking, co-ordination and information sharing between the disabled children's teams, the children's social work teams, complex networks of medical and health services and any relevant adult services (Murray and Osborne 2009: 32). A scoping review by Strathclyde University found that disabled children were seldom involved in child protection conferences and there was little evidence of advocates being used to represent children's views (Stalker et al. 2010). The same finding was evident in a recent Ofsted inspection report which found that even where children communicated well they were not always spoken to directly and advocates were rarely used (2012).

A review of three serious case reviews regarding disabled children highlighted the under-reporting of disabled children in the child protection system and the lack of knowledge and experience of staff working with disabled children (DfES 2006). Abuse is under-reported because of the lack of value placed on disabled children and their relatively powerless position. Oosterhoorn and Kendrick (2001) found that abuse was mainly reported by staff noting physical signs, behaviour or mood changes rather than from a disclosure by the child themselves which highlighted the importance of staff awareness.

In the context of limited resources, disabled children's needs may be seriously neglected as in the second dialogue when the team manager refers to the need for 'strategic reasons' to keep the case as one of *child in need*. It has also been shown that disabled children are neglected through the lack of resources and support services, particularly black and ethnic minority disabled children and their families (NSPCC 2003: 28; Murray and Osborne 2009: 52).

There are barriers for disabled children in accessing protective services. Assessments can become dominated by the child's impairment, social workers can feel limited in expertise and therefore less confident, timescales for assessments do not make allowance for additional time which may be needed and there is a prevalent view that parents are doing their very best for the child (Kitson and Clawson 2007: 173). Edwards and Richardson (2003) also consider that disproportionate weight may be given to medical evidence and that all sources of information must be carefully considered.

Communication: the knowledge base

Knowledge about specific disabilities

Aseem needed to be better informed about Manisha's disability as he would have been in a stronger position to argue for her needs and also to debate issues with the parents and professionals. Although Aseem needed to listen carefully to the parents' views, he also needed to take care as parental accounts can be over-enthusiastic about the child's accomplishments or under-enthusiastic about a child's abilities (Cross et al. 1993: 141). Aseem needed to interrogate the medical jargon and make sure he had an understanding of their communications across agency and professional boundaries. Social workers commonly believe that disabled children do not receive the same protection as non-disabled children because of an unwillingness to recognize abuse and a lack of training (Cooke 2000). Social workers must have an understanding of the nature and impact of various conditions on the child and determine for themselves from the child, family and specialists how the child copes and functions. An NSPCC report (2003: 34) noted that 'child protection workers can sometimes feel out of their depth in terms of knowledge of a child's impairment'.

Manisha's condition, pauciarticular juvenile rheumatoid arthritis is a common form of rheumatoid arthritis mainly affecting girls under the age of eight. It causes inflammation to the knees, elbows, wrists and ankles and may lead to an eye condition iridocyclitis which is potentially a severe complication of the illness. The pain from swollen joints is typically worse in the morning and there may be limited mobility. Besides joint symptoms, the children may have a high fever and a rash which may appear and disappear very quickly. Typically, there are periods when the symptoms can be in remission and times when symptoms flare up. The condition is different in each child.

A child may be unable to describe pain or may become accustomed to the presence of pain. Sometimes children who have repeated medical procedures may be afraid of visits to the doctor which may cause them to not express feelings or identify their pain. A paediatrician and general practitioner frequently manage the treatment of a child often with the help of specialist doctors who may include paediatric rheumatologists, ophthalmologists, sports and exercise physicians, physiotherapists and occupational therapists. The main goals of treatment are to preserve a high level of physical and social functioning and maintain a good quality of life. To achieve these goals, doctors recommend treatments to reduce swelling, maintain full movement in the affected joints, relieve pain, and manage complications.

As well as anti-inflammatory agents such as ibuprofen there are also slower acting agents such as methotrexate. In addition to medications, exercise can help to maintain muscle tone and preserve and recover the range of motion of the joints. The child will have a regular exercise programme and sometimes splints are recommended to keep the joints growing evenly.

Aseem should have been knowledgeable about Manisha's specific medical symptoms and needs. He needed to be familiar with the medical terms and their meaning and to consult with health practitioners in order to become informed. Lack of such knowledge enabled the parents to exert influence on his perceptions and to block his good practice in safeguarding Manisha from harm. Also Aseem had an important role in ensuring the collation of medical information concerning the health needs of Manisha in order to inform the Section 47 investigation (Murray and Osborne 2009: 43).

Legislative and policy framework

The United Nations Convention on the Rights of Persons with Disabilities (2006), enforced in 2008, obliged members to promote equal rights and root out discrimination The rights enshrined in this Convention are the same rights as recognized in the United Nations Convention on the Rights of the Child (1989) with the purpose of promoting, protecting and ensuring the full and equal enjoyment of all human rights and freedoms by all people with disabilities, including children. It includes the right for disabled children to express their views on all issues that affect them and to be protected from violence and abuse. Article 23 concerns the rights of the child to family life and requires states to put in place measures to prevent conceal-ment, abandonment, neglect and segregation (Unicef 2008). The Chronically Sick and Disabled Persons Act 1970 remains a central law for the rights of disabled children and adults in terms of access to services and facilities, including to special education.

The Equality Act 2010 defined a person as having a disability if they have a physical or mental impairment and if the impairment has a substantial and long-term adverse effect on their ability to perform normal day-to-day activities. The Act sought to eliminate discriminatory treatment of disabled children in all areas of public life in the UK including education and provi-sion of services.

The social worker, Aseem, could have used knowledge of legislation and policy guidance to strengthen his arguments with his team manager and to better support the rights of Manisha.

Legislation specifically relevant to this script is Section 17 (Children Act 1989) which states that all disabled child are by definition *children in need*. This imposes a specific duty on local authorities to conduct an assessment of a child's needs. Importantly, an assessment should analyse the child's needs and the parenting capacity, identify whether intervention is needed to secure the child's well-being and lead to a plan of action including the provision of services (DoH 2000: 4.1).

A *child in need* assessment may highlight child protection concerns or allegations about harm may be raised through other sources as in the script where the school staff report concerns about parental neglect of Manisha's needs. 'Disabled children and young people are children first and a disability should not and must not mask or deter an appropriate enquiry where there are child protection concerns' (Murray and Osborne 2009: 13). The national guidance *Safeguarding Disabled Children. Practice Guidance* (Murray and Osborne 2009) provides a framework for collaborative multi-agency child protection responses to safeguard disabled children, including the right to a thorough assessment of their needs and to services to promote their welfare and maximize their independence. This guidance is non-statutory but designed as a supplement to *Working Together to Safeguard Children* (DfE 2010) to ensure that disabled children receive the same level of protection from harm as other children.

Child abuse, disabled children and communication

> I am happy when . . .
> People understand what I am trying to say
> When I talk with people on the same level
> I am happy because I am proud of myself.
> > Kim Goona, 15 yrs (Unicef 2008: 6)

The *Safeguarding Disabled Children* guidance emphasized the 'critical importance of communication with disabled children including recognising that all children can communicate preferences if they are asked in the right way by people who understand their needs and have the skills to listen to them'. It points out that everyone has the right to determine how they wish to describe themselves. In relation to disabled children, for instance, a deaf child may prefer to be regarded as deaf rather than disabled.

If an investigation of significant harm is to be meaningful then 'additional time and resources may need to be allocated' (Murray and Osborne 2009: 36). *Working Together* (DfE 2010: 6.45) emphasized the need to make sure that disabled children communicate their wishes and feelings in respect of their care and treatment and that they know how to raise concerns with a range of adults with whom they can communicate. Barriers that may impede child protection enquiries in relation to communication include the following:

- Judgements about the child's communication not based on specialist advice.
- The child's preferred method of communication is not recognized or equipment/facilitation is not available.
- Augmentative communication systems not containing the words necessary to describe a situation of abuse.

- Insufficient time being given to enable the child to communicate in a full and appropriate manner.
- Independent facilitators and interpreters not being available who are familiar with the child's method of communication (Murray and Osborne 2009: 74).
- It has been noted that social workers are reluctant to engage with disabled children instead preferring to speak with the parents (Stalker et al. 2010: 17).

The family context

In the UK there are 770,000 disabled children under the age of 16 which equates to one child in 20. Of these children 99.1 per cent live at home with their families (Contact a Family 2011a). In *Forgotten Families* (Contact a Family 2011b), the isolation experienced by parents of disabled children is said to lead to break-up in one-fifth of families. Although the families have the 'same hopes and dreams as other families' and 'want to see their children reach their full potential and enjoy time together as a family', they experience an 'overwhelming combination of financial, emotional and practical pressures and without information and support find it difficult to cope and become isolated'. Some isolation resulted from the discrimination and stigma experienced (2011b: 3). Almost three-quarters of families suffered depression and nearly half had relationship difficulties. Over half of the families had financial problems which they linked to the high costs of caring for a disabled child. Aseem needed to have an understanding of the pressures experienced by Manisha's family.

When asked about the most important issues, families said they needed time away from the disabled child and to have a chance to communicate about their problems. Only one in 13 disabled children received any regular support service from their local authority. Although not applicable to the script in this chapter, disabled children are likely to be in poor housing and to be far more likely to grow up in poverty, particularly lone parents, black and ethnic minority families and those with disabled children and parents in the same household (Emerson and Hatton 2005; Beresford and Rhodes 2008; Read et al. 2012: 228).

Disabled children and child protection

It is well reported that disabled children are nearly four times more likely to be physically abused than non-disabled children (Sullivan and Knutson 2000: 1257; Miller 2002) and that the presence of multiple disabilities appears to increase the risk of abuse (DfE 2010: 6.44). An NSPCC study concluded that 'children with special educational needs, long-standing disability or illness . . . were more likely to suffer multiple forms of maltreatment and victimisation' (2011b: 15). Out of a sample of 47 serious case reviews, 5 per cent concerned disabled children with issues mainly relating to neglect and delayed medical treatment which is an over-representation compared with non-disabled children (Brandon et al. 2008: 39). A complex question arising from the association between disability and abuse is causality: 'to what extent does maltreatment contribute to impairment as opposed to disability predisposing to abuse?' (Stalker et al. 2010).

Disabled children are particularly vulnerable to abuse due to their experience of the following:

- Greater social isolation – particularly in institutional care away from their locality making it difficult to be heard or observed by protective adults.
- Greater dependency on others at all ages for personal care, allowing abusers close contact which may not be questioned.
- Increased numbers of carers leading to more potential abusers in the child's world.
- May be unheard when trying to disclose abuse because of communication difficulties or lack of support.
- Abusers target disabled children thinking that the indicators of physical abuse will be misinterpreted as signs of disability and the abuse will remain hidden.
- More vulnerable to abuse by peers.
- May suffer specific forms of physical abuse such as force feeding, excessive physical restraint or rough handling (Davies and Duckett 2008: 130).
- Are particularly vulnerable to bullying and intimidation (DfE 2010: 6.44): 'for many disabled children bullying can be an insidious and relentless pressure that can dominate their lives, leaving them feeling depressed and withdrawn' (Murray and Osborne 2009: 21).

The *London Child Protection Procedures* (LSCB 2010) list the need for professional vigilance relating to specific indicators of abuse in relation to disabled children. These include: force feeding; rough handling; excessive physical restraint; misuse of medication and sedation; extreme behaviour modification including deprivation of liquid, medication, food and clothing; invasive procedures against the child's will; deliberate failure to follow medically recommended regimes; ill-fitting equipment and undignified age or culturally inappropriate intimate care practices. It is important to recognize that some abusive behaviours towards a disabled child may constitute a crime such as inappropriate restraint or intimidation (Murray and Osborne

2009: 37). Relevant to the script in this chapter NSPCC (2003: 33) refer to medication that 'can sometimes be used in ways that can potentially damage the child'.

To ensure equality of access to protection, professionals must be aware of factors which tend to minimize the abuse or lead to denial of, or failure to report, abuse of disabled children. Davies and Ward (2011: 46) state that 'agencies may fail to recognise indicators of neglect in disabled children, or be reluctant to act in the face of concerns'.

While social workers must make sure that the voice of the child is represented through those who know them well, this does not mean that the information obtained is not rigorously assessed and evaluated. Through professionally dangerous practice, social workers may over-sympathize with the family at times leading to collusion and the signs of abuse may become attributed to the disability rather than to neglect. There may be an over-reliance on the main carer for information and it is important to contact a number of different sources to gain a full picture of the child's needs: 'Children are left in situations where there is a high level of neglect . . . because a professional feels the parent, carer or service is doing their best' (NSPCC 2003: 34; Stalker et al. 2010). Social workers may also lack understanding of communication methods and have little knowledge of the child's wishes and feelings and the impact of the disability on their daily lives. They may then also confuse indicators of abuse with behaviours associated with the disability (DfES 2006).

Use of intermediaries

Intermediaries are specialists in assessment of particular communication needs and the skills required relating to a specific child's ability to communicate. The function of an intermediary is to ensure that communication between the child and the criminal justice system is accurate, complete and coherent (Murray and Osborne 2009: 26).

Intermediaries are approved by the court and may be used to help a witness to communicate who has difficulty understanding questions or framing evidence in order to coherently communicate with the court. An intermediary may assist during the investigative interview, during a pre-trial visit and also in court, and must provide written advice to the court explaining relevant communication issues. The intermediary is allowed to explain questions and answers, if that is necessary to enable the witness and the court to communicate. The intermediary does not decide what questions to put. The use of an intermediary does not reduce the responsibility of the judge or magistrates, or of the legal representative, to ensure that the questions put to a witness are proper and appropriate to the level of understanding of the witness (Ministry of Justice 2011: 179).

CASE STUDY AND REFLECTION

A disabled young person unprotected

The striking similarity between Manisha in the script and Damian Clough, in the following case study, is the extent to which they were rendered invisible to decision makers by virtue of their disability. Persistence, therefore, in asserting the rights and entitlements of disabled children is a form of communication critical to both accounts.

In 2009, Damian died age 12 from smoke inhalation after a fire at his home in Keighley, Yorkshire. The family dog was also found dead. The fire was started deliberately, but although two young men stood trial there were no convictions in the case. At the trial his mother said she had left Damian asleep to go to work, that she was mentally tired and had expected his sister back soon.

Damian was autistic, diagnosed as at the severe end of the autistic spectrum. He had some obsessive behaviours such as shredding mattresses and wallpaper. He lived with his mother and sister and had some contact with his father. He was well loved by his family and grandparents and spent one weekend a month in respite care. His parents said they were dominated by him and found it hard to concentrate upon other areas of their lives. Damian had no sense of danger, would run away, would eat anything that he could lay his hands on and break things if left unsupervised. He attended a special school and a respite care unit and professionals in those places also found him difficult to look after. With one-to-one attention in respite care for one weekend every month, his carer was able to look after him and his behaviour when with her was different and much less challenging. The serious case review commented; 'It is clear that the impact of child D's disability on his sister and family was not appropriately considered throughout their lives. This could have been done had the framework for the assessment of children in need and their families been followed, with particular regard to the domain "parenting capacity"' (Raynes 2009: 6.2).

Damian received services throughout his life from different professionals. He attended one school, had an allocated social worker and his case was reviewed every six months. Occupational therapists visited his house and organized adaptations, children's social care provided staff to advise the parents how to look after him and provided respite care in his home and also at the carer's house. Various health services provided assistance with respect to his physical and mental health and a private organization took him out on trips. His sister received services from Barnardo's. Towards the end of Damian's life, his sister was known to social care and police as she was being victimized.

The serious case review (Raynes 2009) concluded: 'There was a sense of tunnel vision in looking to fit Child D's needs into the resources that were available and that all agencies should report child protection concerns and need to be aware of the importance of seeing, speaking to and listening to the child in question . . . staff failed to recognise how at risk the children were because there were no particular events to trigger a child protection investigation' and 'that issues of safeguarding were not considered in the case.'

Questions to aid reflection

Drawing on the knowledge presented in this chapter, and your learning from analysis of the script, consider the following questions:

 How might Aseem have best communicated with Manisha to gain an in-depth understanding of her needs?

 Without having direct contact with Manisha, how did Aseem ensure that she remained central to his work?

 What knowledge base would have assisted Aseem in his persistence to better present Manisha's needs to his manager?

 What pitfalls of professional dangerousness, related to the protection of disabled children, might have distracted Aseem from his persistence in responding to Manisha's needs?

 If Aseem's manager had not listened to his concerns, how might he have taken his analysis of the risks to Manisha further?

Agencies and websites

Social workers need to be informed about the key agencies involved in this area of work so that they know where to access specialist advice and support.

Contact a Family. Website for families with disabled children. http://www. cafamily.org.uk/

Council for Disabled Children. This charity aims to make a difference to the lives of disabled children and children with special educational needs by influencing government policy and producing guidance. http:// councilfordisabledchildren.org.uk/

Don't stick it, stop it! campaign. Campaign against disablist bullying. www. mencap.org.uk

Every Child in Need. Campaign to protect children in need from proposals to change legislation which will be detrimental to their rights and needs. www.everychildinneed.org.uk

Health and Social Care Professionals Council. Registration and standards for social workers and health care professionals. www.hcpc-uk.org

Ofsted whistleblower hotline. Call 0300 123 3155. Email: whistleblowing@ofsted.gov.uk.

Public Concern at Work. Free confidential advice from the independent whistleblowing charity. Call 020 7404 6609. www.pcaw.org

Resources

How It Is. This consists of an image vocabulary for children about feelings, rights and safety, personal care and sexuality. It consists of 380 images designed to support children communicating about their feelings, bodies, rights and basic needs. http://www.howitis.org.uk/browse_p5.htm

In My Shoes. A computer-assisted approach to the investigative interviewing of children and vulnerable adults. This resource can be used for assessment and therapeutic interviews. It may also be used in conducting or preparing for an ABE interview. It is particularly useful for young people and children who may have difficulty in expressing emotions (and may not use the spoken word) or have developmental delay. www.inmyshoes.org.uk

My Life, My Decisions, My Choice. A set of resources to aid decision-making. It includes a poster, discussion cards and a guide for professionals. http://sites.childrenssociety.org.uk/disabilitytoolkit/about/resources.aspx

***Other Ways of Speaking:* Supporting Children and Young People who have no Speech or whose Speech is Difficult to Understand (Communication Trust 2011).** This booklet explores augmentative and alternative communication (AAC), a term which describes a wide range of techniques children and young people use to support or replace spoken communication. http://www.thecommunicationtrust.org.uk/media/3414/other_ways_of_speaking_final.pdf

Talking Mats. Communication tool using mats with symbols attached as basis for communication. www.talkingmats.com

Two-Way Street: Communication with Disabled Children and Young People (Triangle 2001). Training dvd and handbook. www.triangle-services.co.uk/index.php?page=publications

Recommended reading

Calder, M. (2008) Organisational dangerousness: causes, consequences and correctives, in M. Calder (ed.) *Contemporary Risk Assessment in Safeguarding Children*. Lyme Regis: Russell House.

DfES (Department of Education and Skills, 2006) *Safeguarding Disabled Children: A Resource for Local Safeguarding Children Boards*. London: DfES.

Kline, R. and Preston-Shoot, M. (2012) *Professional Accountability in Social Care and Health: Challenging Unacceptable Practice and its Management*. London: Learning Matters.

Murray, M. and Osborne, C. (2009) *Safeguarding Disabled Children: Practice Guidance*. London: Department of Children, Schools and Families.

Ofsted (2012) *Protecting Disabled Children*. Available from: http://www.ofsted.gov.uk/resources/protecting-disabled-children-thematic-inspection [Accessed 22 November 2012].

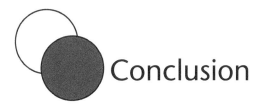 Conclusion

In writing this book the authors have, through five scripts, brought to life examples of current, relevant and contested areas of social work. These have been explored through five key aspects of communication – engagement, negotiation, investigation, use of power and persistence – and presented in a context of broad aspects of good professional practice. The current relevance of the scripts has been given weight through comparison with a contemporary case study. Each chapter has presented practice means of assisting social workers to explore finding the *power with* children and families and the *power to* challenge childism at every level of their work.

As the enormity of crimes committed against children becomes increasingly under the media, political and public spotlight, the social work role in communicating effectively with children and young people becomes more important than ever (http://spotlightonabuse.wordpress.com). Survivors commonly speak of the one social worker who listened to them as being key to their healing. They also describe social workers who for whatever reason did not protect them and did not listen as being complicit in the abuse. In all situations of crime committed against children there are those who perpetrate the crimes, those who collude with the perpetrators and facilitate the abuse, those who knowingly or unknowingly support the perpetrators by not challenging or reporting the abuse, and finally those who, through ignorance and incompetence, just do not understand or recognize the crimes being committed in front of them and do not hear children's voices. In serious case reviews, the actual words of the children who have been harmed or who died have rarely been evident. It is indicative of seriously flawed social work communication practice that the child's own views and perspectives were rarely heard or represented.

Social work with children and young people carries with it major responsibilities. It is important to read about social workers who have truly made a difference and retained their professional integrity and authenticity when under pressure to conceal the truth about harm to children or when bearing witness to injustice. Social worker Margaret Humphreys noted from one interview with one adult who had been adopted in childhood that there must have been more cases and this led her to bravely expose the post-war scandal of the child migrants. These were children trafficked in their thousands from children's homes in the UK, by charities supported by the government, to Australia and Canada to provide a workforce in those countries (Humphreys 2011). Alison Taylor, a social worker in North Wales, helped to expose extensive crimes committed against children in the residential system: 'a number of other social workers managed to live with it. One said to me that if I said something I'd be committing professional suicide. But if I come across something morally wrong, I can't leave it. I thought sooner or later someone had to stand up and be counted' (Morrison 2012). Nevres Kemal, a former social worker in Haringey Children's Services, alerted management to flaws in the child protection systems. She said: 'I never regretted speaking up for the children who needed protection . . . I never thought, even when I was at my most scared, why did I not keep my mouth shut? You can take everything from me: my home, my job, my good name but you cannot strip me of my integrity' (Fairweather 2008c). Simon Bellwood, a social worker in Jersey, raised the alarm about mistreatment of young people. He reported a 'Dickensian' system in a secure unit where children as young as 11 were routinely locked up for 24 hours or more in solitary confinement. He said: 'It has never been about me. If it were, then I would have been better off keeping my mouth shut and my head down all these past months. I just want justice for these children who deserve a better deal than the one they are currently enduring' (Ahmed 2007). These social workers had personal and professional awareness of the political and social context of their work situation and made use of their skills in social activism to achieve change and challenge the oppression of children – childism.

Everyday events in the working life of a social worker may be indicative of wider issues of social oppression but social workers cannot always see the bigger picture. However, they must strive to be well informed, have a strong knowledge base and retain rigorous professional standards, values and ethics. This is the meaning of professional accountability to the service user, the public interest and the profession as outlined in the Introduction. This role will not be achievable without multi-agency working and close liaison by social workers with service user groups and campaign organizations. Authentic social workers also need to work within safe environments with quality training and supervision, reasonable caseloads and responsible supportive management. If they feel helpless to address their own poor work conditions then social workers will struggle to represent the interests of service users.

Through the writing of this book, the authors hope to enter into dialogue with the reader leading to a positive impact on social work practice. It is intended that the book will promote understanding about the complex, specialist nature of social work with children and their families and support a profession skilled in representing the best interests of children and young people, responding to their needs and protecting them from harm.

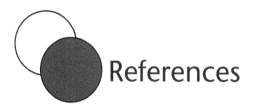

References

Adcock, M. and White, R. (1998) *Significant Harm: Its Management and Outcome*. London: Significant Publications.

Ahmed, M. (2007) Social worker blows the whistle on Jersey, *Community Care*, 7 September.

Aldridge, M. and Wood, J. (1998) *Interviewing Children: A Guide for Child Care and Forensic Practitioners*. Chichester: Wiley.

Alexander, S.M., Baur, L.A., Magnusson, R. and Tobin, B. (2009) When does severe childhood obesity become a child protection issue?, *Medical Journal of Australia*, 190: 136–139.

Alinsky, S. (1969) *Reveille for Radicals*. New York: Vintage.

Alinsky, S. (1971) *Rules for Radicals*. New York: Vintage.

Allen, G. and Langford, D. (2008) *Effective Interviewing in Social Work and Social Care*. Basingstoke: Palgrave Macmillan.

Aylott, J., Brown, I., Copeland, R. and Johnson, D. (2008) *Tackling Obesities: The Foresight Report and Implications for Local Government*. Sheffield: Sheffield Hallam University.

Banks, S. (2004) *Ethics, Accountability and the Social Professions*. Basingstoke: Palgrave Macmillan.

Banks, S. (2010) Integrity in professional life: issues of conduct, commitment and capacity, *British Journal of Social Work*, 40: 2168–2184.

Barker, J. and Hodes D. (2007) *A Child in Mind*. London: Routledge.

BASW (British Association of Social Workers, 2012a) *A Code of Ethics for Social Work*. Available from: http://cdn.basw.co.uk/upload/basw_112315–7.pdf [Accessed 21 November 2012].

BASW (British Association of Social Workers, 2012b) *The State of Social Work*. Available from: http://cdn.basw.co.uk/upload/basw_23651–3.pdf [Accessed 21 November 2012].

Beresford, B. and Rhodes, D. (2008) *Housing and Disabled Children*. York: Joseph Rowntree Foundation.

Bhabha, J. and Finch, N. (2006) *Seeking Asylum Alone*. London: Harvard University Committee on Human Rights Studies.

Blackwell, D. and Melzak, S. (2000) *Far from the Battle but still at War: Troubled Refugee Children at School*. London: Psychotherapy Trust.

Blaug, R. (1995) Distortion of the face to face: communicative reasoning and social work practice, *British Journal of Social Work*, 25: 423–439.

Boylan, J. and Dalrymple, J. (2009) *Understanding Advocacy for Children and Young People*. Maidenhead: Open University Press.

Brandon, M. (2002) *Overview Report Concerning the Case of Lauren Wright*. Norfolk: Norfolk Social Services Department.

Brandon, M., Balderson, P., Warren, C., Howe, D., Gardner, R., Dodsworth, D. and Black, J. (2008) *Analysing Child Deaths and Serious Injury through Abuse and Neglect: What Can We Learn?* London: Department of Children Schools and Families.

Briggs, S. (2008) *Working with Adolescents and Young Adults: A Contemporary Psychodynamic Approach*. Basingstoke: Palgrave Macmillan.

Broadhurst, K., Grover, C. and Jamieson, J. (eds) (2009) *Critical Perspectives on Safeguarding Children*. Chichester: Wiley.

Brownlees, L. and Finch, N. (2010) *Levelling the Playing Field: A UNICEF Report into Provision of Services to Unaccompanied or Separated Migrant Children in Three Local Authority Areas in England*. London: UNICEF.

Burdett, J. (2010) *State Sponsored Cruelty: Children in Immigration Centres*. London: Medical Justice.

Burke, C. (1994) *Being an Effective Advocate for the Child: Children who Experience Domestic Violence*. Sydney: New South Wales Child Protection Council.

Calder, M. (ed.) (2008) *Contemporary Risk Assessment in Safeguarding Children*. Lyme Regis: Russell House.

Calder, M. (2008) Organisational dangerousness: causes, consequences and correctives, in M. Calder (ed.) *Contemporary Risk Assessment in Safeguarding Children*. Lyme Regis: Russell House.

Calder, M. and Hackett, S. (eds) (2003) *Assessment in Child Care*. Lyme Regis: Russell House.

Camden Area Child Protection Committee (ACPC) (2004) *Children Abused Through Sexual Exploitation: Policy and Guidance*. London: Camden ACPC.

Chamba, R., Ahmad, W., Hirst, M., Lawton, D. and Beresford, B. (1999) *On the Edge: Minority Ethnic Families Caring for a Severely Disabled Child*. Bristol: The Policy Press.

Chamberlain, P. (2007) Tell it like it is, *Community Care*, 5–11 April: 24–25.

Children's Society (2008) *Give Me a Life: Personal Testimonies by Children Seeking Asylum in the UK*. DVD available from: www.societyofeditors.org.

Children's Society (2011a) Almost 700 children detained in three months. Press release, 17 October. Available from: http://www.childrenssociety.org.uk/news-views/press-release/almost–700-children-detained-four-months [Accessed 22 November 2012].

Children's Society (2011b) *What Have I Done? The Experience of Children and Families in UK Immigration Detention: Lessons to Learn*. London: Children's Society.

Cleaver, H. and Nicholson, D. (2007) *Parental Learning Disability and Children's Needs: Family Experiences and Effective Practice.* London: Jessica Kingsley Publishers.

College of Social Work (2012) *The Professional Capabilities Framework.* Available from: http://www.collegeofsocialwork.org/pcf.aspx [Accessed 22 November 2012].

Contact a Family (2011a) Facts and statistics. Available from: http://www.cafamily.org.uk/professionals/research [Accessed 21 November 2012].

Contact a Family (2011b) *Forgotten Families: The Impact of Isolation on Families with Disabled Children across the UK.* London: Contact a Family.

Cooke, P. (2000) *Final Report on Disabled Children and Abuse – Research Project.* Nottingham: Ann Craft Trust.

Cossar, A., Brandon, M. and Jordan, P. (2011) *'Don't Make Assumptions': Children's and Young People's Views of the Child Protection System and Messages for Change.* London: Office of the Children's Commissioner.

Council of Europe (1950) *European Convention for the Protection of Human Rights and Fundamental Freedoms*, 4 November 1950. Available from: http://www.unhcr.org/refworld/docid/3ae6b3b04.html [Accessed 21 November 2012].

CQC (Care Quality Commission, 2009) *Review of the Involvement and Action taken by Health Bodies in the Case of Baby P.* London: CQC.

CRAE (Children's Rights Alliance England, 2011) *The State of Children's Rights in England.* London: CRAE.

Crawley, H. (2012) *Working with Children and Young People subject to Immigration Control. Guidelines for Best Practice, 2nd edn.* London: Immigration Law Practitioners' Association.

Cross, M., Gordon, R., Kennedy, M. and Marchant, R. (1993) *The ABCD Pack. Abuse and Children who are Disabled.* Leicester: NSPCC.

Daniel, B., Wassell, S. and Gilligan, R. (1999) *Child Development for Child Care and Protection Workers.* London: Jessica Kingsley Publishers.

Davidson, J. and Gottschalk, P. (eds) (2011) *Internet Child Abuse: Current Research and Policy.* London: Routledge.

Davies, C. and Ward, H. (2011) *Safeguarding Children across Services: Messages from Research.* London: Jessica Kingsley Publishers.

Davies, G. and Westcott, H. (1999) *Interviewing Child Witnesses under the Memorandum of Good Practice: A Research Review.* London: Home Office.

Davies, L. (2006) Responding to the protection needs of traumatized sexually abused children, in A. Hosin (ed.) *Responses to Traumatised Children.* Basingstoke: Palgrave Macmillan.

Davies, L. (2008a) Where next for social work?, *Professional Social Work*, December.

Davies, L. (2008b) *Reforms have been imposed at the expense of protecting children*, Society Guardian online. 2 December.

Davies, L. (2009) Let's get rid of social work's blame culture, Society Guardian online. 25 June.

Davies, L. and Duckett, N. (2008) *Proactive Child Protection and Social Work*. London: Learning Matters.

Davies, L. and Townsend, D. (2008) *Working Together, Training Together: Achieving Best Evidence*. Lyme Regis: Russell House.

DCSF (Department of Children, Schools and Families, 2009) *Safeguarding Children and Young People from Sexual Exploitation: Supplementary Guidance to Working Together*. London: The Stationery Office

Derby Safeguarding Children Board (2010) *Serious Case Review BD09 Executive Summary*. Derby: Derby Safeguarding Children Board.

DfE (Department for Education, 2010) *Working Together to Safeguard Children: A Guide to Inter-agency Working to Safeguard and Promote the Welfare of Children*. London: The Stationery Office.

DfE (Department for Education, 2012) *What to Do if You Suspect a Child is being Sexually Exploited: A Step-by-step Guide for Frontline Practitioners*. London: The Stationery Office.

DfES (Department for Education and Skills, 2006) *Safeguarding Disabled Children: A Resource for Local Safeguarding Children Boards*. London: DfES.

DHSS (Department of Health and Social Security, 1988) *Working Together: A Guide to Arrangements for Inter-agency Cooperation for the Protection of Children from Abuse*. London: HMSO.

DoH (Department of Health, 1989) *The Children Act*. London: The Stationery Office.

DoH (Department of Health, 2000) *Framework of Assessment for Children in Need and their Families*. London: The Stationery Office.

DoH/DfES Department of Health and Department for Education and Skills, 2006) *Good Practice Guidance on Working with Parents with a Learning Disability*. London: Department of Health.

Donnelly, L. (2011) Obesity crisis: half a million children have liver disease, *The Telegraph,* 3 July.

ECPAT UK (2011) *Briefing: Guardianship for Child Victims of Trafficking*. Available from: www.ecpat.org.uk/sites/default/files/guardianship_briefing.pdf [Accessed 22 November 2012].

Edwards, H. and Richardson, K. (2003) The child protection system and disabled children, in NSPCC *It Doesn't Happen to Disabled Children*. London: NSPCC.

Emerson, E. and Hatton, C. (2005) *The Socio-economic Circumstances of Families Supporting a Child at Risk of Disability in Britian in 2002*. Lancaster: Institute for Health Research.

England, H. (1986) *Social Work as Art*. London: HarperCollins.

Fairweather, E. (1998) The Islington child abuse scandal, in G. Hunt (ed.) *Whistleblowing in the Social Services: Public Accountability and Professional Practice*. London: Hodder Arnold.

Fairweather, E. (2008a) Revealed: how a close male relative of Baby P is linked to a big paedophile network, *Daily Mail*, 16 November.

Fairweather, E. (2008b) Baby P relative implicated in child sex ring, *Sunday Times*, 14 December.

Fairweather, E. (2008c) Baby P council falsely accused me of abusing a child, reveals whistleblower who feared she'd lose her daughter, Mail on Sunday, 16 November.

Ferguson, H. (2004) *Protecting Children in Time: Child Abuse, Child Protection and the Consequences of Modernity*. Basingstoke: Palgrave Macmillan.

Ferguson, H. (2011) *Child Protection Practice*. Basingstoke: Palgrave Macmillan.

Fisher, D. and Gruescu, S. (2011) *Children and the Big Society*. London: Action for Children.

Fletcher, K. (1998) *Negotiation for Health and Social Services Professional*. London: Jessica Kingsley Publishers.

Foley, P. and Rixon, A. (eds) (2008) *Changing Children's Services Working and Learning Together*. Bristol: The Policy Press.

Fonagy, P. and Target, M. (1997) Attachment and reflective function: their role in self-organization, *Development and Psychopathology*, 9: 679–700.

Fook, J. (2002) *Social Work Critical Theory and Practice*. London: Sage.

Fook, J. and Askeland, G. A. (2007) Challenges of critical reflection: 'nothing ventured, nothing gained', *Social Work Education*, 16(2): 1–14.

Frampton, P. (2009) Lecture at London Metropolitan University, 11 December.

Friere, P. (1972) *Pedagogy of the Oppressed*. London: Penguin.

Frost, N. (2005) *Professionalism, Partnership and Joined-up Thinking*. Darlington: Research in Practice.

Garrett, P. (2003a) *Remaking Social Work with Children and Families: A Critical Discussion on the Modernisation of Social Care*. London: Routledge.

Garrett, P. (2003b) Swimming with dolphins: the assessment framework, New Labour and new tools for social work with children and families, *British Journal of Social Work*, 33: 441–463.

Gillen, S. (2002) Independent comment, *Community Care*, 17 April: 18.

Glenny, G. and Roaf, C. (2008) *Multiprofessional Communication: Making Systems Work for Children*. Maidenhead: Open University Press.

Goleman, D. (1996) *Emotional Intelligence*. London: Bloomsbury.

Gregory, M. and Holloway, M. (2005) Language and the shaping of social work, *British Journal of Social Work*, 35: 37–53.

Griffiths, J. (2010) Is obesity a child protection issue? *Community Care*, 9 January.

Habermas, J. (1976) *Legitimation Crisis*. Cambridge: Polity Press.

Hackett, S. (2003) A framework for assessing parenting capacity, in M. Calder and S. Hackett (eds) *Assessment in Child Care*. Lyme Regis: Russell House.

Harris, P. and Bright, M. (2003) The whistleblower's story, *The Guardian*, 6 July. Available from: http://www.guardian.co.uk/politics/2003/jul/06/children.childprotection [Accessed 12 July 2012].

HCPC (Health and Care Professions Council, 2012a) *How to Raise and Escalate a Concern*. Available from: http://www.hpc-uk.org/registrants/raisingconcerns/howto/ [Accessed 22 November 2012].

HCPC (Health and Care Professions Council, 2012b) *Whistleblowing*. Available from: http://www.hpc-uk.org/registrants/raisingconcerns/whistleblowing/ [Accessed 22 November 2012].

HCPC (Health and Care Professionals Council, 2012c) *Mapping of the HCPC Standards of Proficiency for Social Workers in England with the Professional Capabilities Framework (PCF)*. Available from: http://www.hpc-uk.org/assets/documents/10003B0BMappingoftheHPC'sstandardsofproficiencyforsocialworkersinEngland [Accessed 22 November 2012].

Hek, R. (2007) Using foster placements for the care and resettlement of unaccompanied children, in R. Kohli and F. Mitchell (eds) *Working with Unaccompanied Asylum Seeking children: Issues for Policy and Practice*. Basingstoke: Palgrave Macmillan.

HLSCB (Haringey Local Safeguarding Children Board, 2008) *Support Offered to Family of Child A: Document within Serious Case Review Executive Summary*. London: HLSCB.

HLSCB (Haringey Local Safeguarding Children Board, 2009) *Serious Case Review: Baby Peter. Executive Summary*. London: HLSCB.

HMIP (Her Majesty's Inspector of Prisons, 2011) *Three Reports on Unannounced Inspections of the Short Term Holding Facility at Heathrow Airport Terminal 1, 3 and 4 (March–April)*. London: HMIP.

Home Office (2004) *Protecting the Public from Sexual Crime – An Explanation of the Sexual Offences Act 2003*. London: Home Office.

Home Office (2009) *Every Child Matters: Change for Children. Statutory Guidance to the UK Border Agency on Making Arrangements to Safeguard and Promote the Welfare of Children*. London: Home Office and Department for Children, Schools and Families.

Home Office (2011) *Immigration Statistics*. Available from: http://www.homeoffice.gov.uk/publications/science-research-statistics/research-statistics/immigration-asylum-research/immigration-brief-q2–2011/asylum [Accessed 12 July 2012].

Howe, D. (1996) Surface and depth in social work practice, in N. Parton (ed.) *Social Work Theory, Social Change and Social Work*. London: Routledge.

Howe, D. (2008) *The Emotionally Intelligent Social Worker*. Basingstoke: Palgrave Macmillan.

Howe, D. (2009) *A Brief Introduction to Social Work Theory*. Basingstoke: Palgrave Macmillan.

Humphreys, M. (2011) *Oranges and Sunshine: Empty Cradles*. London. Corgi.

IFSW (International Federation of Social Work, 2012) *Statement of Ethical Principles*. Available from: http://ifsw.org/policies/statement-of-ethical-principles [Accessed 22 November 2012].

Interpol (2011) *Blocking Access to Child Abuse images*. Available from: http://www.interpol.int/Public/THBInternetAccessBlocking/Terminology.asp [Accessed 2 July 2011].

IWF (Internet Watch Foundation, 2008) *UK Adult Internet Users.2008 Research Report*. Available from: https://www.iwf.org.uk/assets/media/news/IWF%20UK%20Adult%20Internet%20Users%20Survey%202008.pdf [Accessed 22 November 2012].

James, H. (2010) Supporting parents with a learning disability, *Learning Disability Practice*, 13: 12–17.

Jones, M. (2011) Delays in paedophile database putting children at risk. BBC Newsnight: Available from: http://news.bbc.co.uk/1/mobile/programmes/newsnight/9532058.stm [Accessed 22 November 2012].

Kennedy, M. and Wonnacott, J. (2003) Disabled children and the assessment framework, in M. Calder and S. Hackett (eds) *Assessment in Child Care*. Lyme Regis: Russell House.

Kerrigan Lebloch, E. and King, S (2006) Child sexual exploitation: a partnership response and model intervention, *Child Abuse Review*, 15(5): 362–372.

Kitson, D. and Clawson, R. (2007) Safeguarding children with disabilities, in K. Wilson and A. James (eds) *The Child Protection Handbook*. London: Elsevier.

Kline, R. (2010) *What if? Social Care Professionals and the Duty of Care: A Practical Guide to Staff Duties and Rights*. London: Aspect (Association of Professionals in Education and Children's Trusts).

Kline, R. and Preston-Shoot, M. (2012) *Professional Accountability in Social Care and Health: Challenging Unacceptable Practice and its Management*. London: Learning Matters.

Kohli, R. (2006) The sound of silence: listening to what unaccompanied asylum seeking children say and do not say, *British Journal of Social Work*, 36: 707–721.

Kohli, R. (2007) *Social Work with Unaccompanied Asylum Seeking Children*. Basingstoke: Palgrave Macmillan.

Kohli, R. (2011) Working to ensure safety, belonging and success for unaccompanied, asylum seeking children, *Child Abuse Review*, 20: 311–323.

Kohli, R. and Mather, R. (2003) Promoting psychosocial well-being in unaccompanied asylum seeking young people in the United Kingdom, *Child and Family Social Work*, 8: 201–212.

Kohli, R. and Mitchell, F. (eds) (2007) *Working with Unaccompanied Asylum Seeking Children: Issues for Policy and Practice*. Basingstoke: Palgrave Macmillan.

Koprowska, J. (2007) *Communication and Interpersonal Skills in Social Work*. Exeter: Learning Matters.

Laming, H. (2003) *The Victoria Climbié Inquiry Report*. London: The Stationery Office.

Lasswell, H. (1948) The structure and function of communication in society, in L. Bryson (ed.) *The Communication of Ideas*. New York: Harper and Row.

Lefevre, M. (2010) *Communicating with Children and Young People: Making a Difference.* Bristol: The Policy Press.

Lepper, J. (2012) Disabled children are overlooked by child protection services, *Children and Young People Now*, 22 August.

Lishman, J. (1993) *Communication in Social Work.* Basingstoke: Palgrave Macmillan.

Lorek, A., Ehntholt, K., Nesbitt, A., Wey, E., Githinji, C., Rossor, E. and Wickramasinghe, R. (2009) The mental and physical health difficulties of children held within a British immigration detention centre, *Child Abuse and Neglect*, 33: 573–585.

LSCB (London Safeguarding Children Board, 2010) *London Child Protection Procedures.* London: LSCB.

Luft, J. and Ingham, H. (2007). The Johari window: a graphic model of interpersonal awareness, in M. Lymbery and K. Postle (eds) *Social Work: A Companion to Learning.* London: Sage.

Lymbery, M. and Butler, S. (2004) *Social Work Ideals and Practice Realities.* Basingstoke: Palgrave Macmillan.

Lymbery, M. and Postle, K. (2007) *Social Work: A Companion to Learning.* London: Sage.

McGaw, S. and Newman, T. (2005) *What Works for Parents with Learning Disabilities?* Basildon: Barnardo's.

Matthews, A. (2011) *Landing in Kent: The Experience of Unaccompanied Children Arriving in the UK.* London: Office of the Children's Commissioner.

Melrose, M. and Barrett, D. (eds) (2004) *Anchors in Floating Lives: Inteviews with Young People Sexually Abused through Prostitution.* Lyme Regis: Russell House.

Mepham, S. (2010) Disabled children: the right to feel safe, *Child Care in Practice*, 16(1): 19–34.

Miller, D. (2002) *Disabled Children and Abuse.* Available from: http://www.nspcc.org.uk/Inform/research/Briefings/disabledchildrenandabuse_wda48224.html [Accessed 22 November 2012].

Ministry of Justice (2011) *Achieving Best Evidence in Criminal Proceedings: Guidance on Vulnerable or Intimidated Witnesses, including Children.* London: Ministry of Justice.

Mitchell, K., Finkelhor, D. and Wolak, J. (2005) The internet and family and acquaintance sexual abuse, *Child Maltreatment*, 10(1): 49–60.

Morley, I. (2006) Negotiation and bargaining, in O. Hargie (ed.) *Handbook of Communication Skills.* London: Routledge.

Morris, K. (2008) *Social Work and Multi-agency Working: Making a Difference.* Bristol: The Policy Press.

Morrison, S. (2012) Woman who blew whistle on abuse breaks her silence, *Independent on Sunday*, 25 November, p. 17.

Morrison, T. (1998) Partnership, collaboration and change under the Children Act, in M. Adcock, and R. White (eds) *Significant Harm: Its Management and Outcome.* Croydon: Significant Publications.

Morrison, T. (2000) Working together to safeguard children: challenges and changes for inter-agency co-ordination in child protection, *Journal of Interprofessional Care*, 14(4): 363–373.

Morrison, T. (2007) Emotional intelligence, emotion and social work: context, characteristics, complications and contribution, *British Journal of Social Work*, 37(2): 245–263.

Mougne, C. (2010) *Trees Only Move in the Wind: A Study of Unaccompanied Afghan Children in Europe*. Geneva: UN Refugee Agency.

Munro, E. (1999) Common errors of reasoning in child protection work, *Child Abuse and Neglect*, 223: 745–758.

Munro, E. (2003) *Effective Child Protection*. London: Sage.

Munro, E. (2008) *Effective Child Protection*, 2nd edn. London: Sage.

Munro, E. (2011) *The Munro Review of Child Protection. Final Report: A Child-centered System*. London: DfE.

Munro, E. and Calder, M. (2005) Where has child protection gone?, *Political Quarterly*, 76(3): 439–445.

Murray, M. and Osborne, C. (2009) *Safeguarding Disabled Children: Practice Guidance*. London: Department of Children, Schools and Families.

Nelson, S. (2007) *See Us-Hear Us: Schools Working with Sexually Abused Young People*. Dundee: Violence is Preventable.

NPIA (National Policing Improvement Agency, 2009) *Guidance on Investigating Child Abuse and Safeguarding Children*, 2nd edn. London: NPIA.

NSPCC (National Society for the Prevention of Cruelty to Children, 2003) *'It Doesn't Happen to Disabled Children': Child Protection and Disabled Children. Report of the National Working Group on Child Protection and Disability*. London: NSPCC.

NSPCC (2008) *Policy Summary: Child Abuse Images*. Available from: http://www.nspcc.org.uk/Inform/policyandpublicaffairs/policysummaries/childabuse-images_wdf56933.pdf [Accessed 7 July 2011].

NSPCC (2010) *Snapshot of Court Cases reveals 2 million Online Child Sexual Abuse Images*. Available from: http://www.nspcc.org.uk/news-and-views/media-centre/press-releases/2010/10–04–28-court-case-reveals–2m-online-child-sex-abuse-images/10–04–28-NSPCC_snapshot_of_court_cases_reveals_2m_online_child_sex_abuse_images_wdn76857.html [Accessed 7 July 2011].

NSPCC (2011a) *All Babies Count*. Available from: http://allbabiescount.nspcc.org.uk [Accessed 6 January 2012].

NSPCC (2011b) *Child Cruelty in the UK 2011: An NSPCC Study into Childhood Abuse and Neglect over the past 30 Years*. London: NSPCC.

NSPCC (2011c) *Child Homicides: Key Child Protection Statistics*. Available from: http://www.nspcc.org.uk/inform/research/statistics/child_homicide_statis-tics_wda48747.html [Accessed 11 July 2011].

OCC (Office of the Children's Commissioner, 2006) *Bullying Today: A Report*. London: OCC.

Ofsted (2011) *The Voice of the Child: Learning Lessons from Serious Case Reviews. A Thematic Report of Ofsted's Evaluation of Serious Case Reviews from 1 April to 30 September 2010*. Manchester: Ofsted.

Ofsted (2012) *Protecting Disabled Children*. Available from: http://www.ofsted.gov.uk/resources/protecting-disabled-children-thematic-inspection. [Accessed 22 November 2012].

Ofsted, Healthcare Commission and HM Inspectorate of Constabulary (2008) *Joint Area Review. Haringey Children's Services Authority Area: Review of Services for Children and Young People, with particular reference to Safeguarding*. London: Ofsted.

Okitikpi, T. (ed.) (2011) *Social Control and the Use of Power in Social Work with Children and Families*. Lyme Regis: Russell House.

Oosterhoorn, R. and Kendrick, A. (2001) No sign of harm: issues for disabled children communicating about abuse, *Child Abuse Review*, 10: 243–253.

Owen, H. and Pritchard, L. (eds) (1993) *Good Practice in Child Protection: A Manual for Professionals*. London: Jessica Kingsley Publishers.

Parrish, M. (2010) *Social Work Perspectives on Human Behaviour*. Maidenhead: Open University Press.

Parton, N. (2006) *Safeguarding Childhood: Early Intervention and Surveillance in Late Modern Society*. Basingstoke: Palgrave Macmillan.

Parton, N. (2008) Changes in the form of knowledge of social work: from the social to the informational, *British Journal of Social Work*, 38: 253–269.

Raynes, B. (2009) *Serious Case Review Executive Summary: Child D. Born 27 May 1996. Died 4th April 2009*. Bradford: Bradford Local Safeguarding Children Board. Available from: http://bradford-scb.org.uk/PDF/Child_D_exec_summary020211.pdf.

Read, J., Blackburn, C. and Spencer, N. (2012) Disabled children and their families: a decade of policy change, *Children and Society*, 26: 223–233.

Reder, P. and Duncan, S. (2003) Understanding communication in child protection networks, *Child Abuse Review*, 12: 82–100.

Reder, P., Duncan, S. and Gray, M. (1993) *Beyond Blame: Child Abuse Tragedies Revisited*. London: Routledge.

RBSCB (Rochdale Borough Safeguarding Children Board, 2012) *Review of Multi-agency Responses to the Sexual Exploitation of Children*. Rochdale: RBSCB.

RCC (Refugee Children's Consortium, 2011) *Memorandum of Evidence to the Education Select Committee on the Inquiry into the Child Protection System in England*. Available from: http://www.childrenssociety.org.uk/sites/default/files/tcs/u32/rcc_submission_to_the_child_protection_inquiry_-_october_2011_2.pdf [Accessed 22 November 2012].

RMJ (Refugee and Migrant Justice, 2009) *Does Every Child Matter?* London: RMJ.

RMJ (Refugee and Migrant Justic, 2010) *Safe at Last? Children on the Front Line of UK Border Control*. London: RMJ.

Saunders, B. and Goddard, C. (2010) *Physical Punishment in Childhood: The Rights of the Child.* Chicheste: Wiley.

Save the Children (2006) *Visible Evidence – Forgotten Children.* Brussels: Save the Children.

Schon, D. (1983) *The Reflective Practitioner.* New York: Basic Books.

Shannon, C. and Weaver, W. (1964) *The Mathematical Theory of Communication.* Urbana, IL: University of Illinois Press.

Shennan, G. (2006) Doing it in child protection, *Solution News*, 2(3).

Sheridan, M. (2008) *From Birth to Five Years: Children's Developmental Progress, 3rd edn.* London: Routledge.

Singh, R. (2009) Social services involved in the Baby P child cruelty case ignored 60 other children in danger, *Evening Standard*, 14 April.

Sirriyeh, A. (2010) Unicef UK research into the experiences of unaccompanied asylum seeking children, *Community Care*, 24 June.

Sirriyeh, A. (2011) Research: good practice when working with refugee and asylum-seeking children, *Community Care*, 15 April.

Sjoberg, R. L. and Lindblad, F. (2003) Limited disclosure of sexual abuse in children whose experiences were documented by videotape, *American Journal of Psychiatry*, 159(2): 312–314.

Smale, G., Tucson, G. and Statham, D. (2000) *Social Work and Social Problems.* Basingstoke: Palgrave Macmillan.

Smith, C. (2001) Trust and confidence: possibilities for social work in 'high modernity', *British Journal of Social Work*, 31: 287–305.

Smith, C. (2004) Trust and confidence: making the moral case for social work, *Social Work and Social Services Review*, 11(3): 287–306.

Social Work Reform Board (2011) *Standards for Employers of Social Workers in England and Supervision Framework.* Available from: http://www.education.gov.uk/swrb/a0074263/standards-for-employers-and-supervision-framework [Accessed 21 November 2012].

Spandler, H. (1996) *Who's Hurting Who? Young People, Self-harm and Suicide.* Manchester: 42nd Street.

Stalker, K., Green Lister, P., Lerpiniere, J. and McArthur, K. (2010) *Child Protection and the Needs and Rights of Disabled Children and Young People: A Scoping Study.* Glasgow: University of Strathclyde.

Steinberg, L. (1993) *Adolescence.* Maidenhead: McGraw-Hill.

Stop it Now (2005) *The Internet and Children – What's the Problem?* London: Stop it Now.

Sullivan, P. and Knutson, J. (2000) Maltreatment and disabilities, *Child Abuse and Neglect*, 24(10): 1257–1273.

Summitt, R. (1983) The child abuse accommodation syndrome, *Child Abuse and Neglect*, 7: 177–193.

Svedin, C. G. and Bach, K. (1997) *Children Who Don't Speak Out: About Children being Used in Child Pornography.* London: Jessica Kingsley Publishers.

Swann, S., McNosh, D. and Edwards, S. (1998) *Whose Daughter Next: Children Abused through Prostitution*. Basildon: Barnardo's.

Taylor, A. (2003) *Responding to Adolescents: Helping Relationship Skills for Youth Workers, Mentors and other Advisors*. Lyme Regis: Russell House.

Taylor, R. C. (2006) Narrating significant experience: reflective accounts and the production of(self) knowledge, *British Journal of Social Work*, 36: 189–206.

Taylor, M. and Quayle, E. (2003) *Child Pornography: An Internet Crime*. London. Routledge.

Taylor-Brown, J. (2002) *More Than One Chance! Young People Involved in Prostitution Speak Out*. London: National Children Homes, DoH, Home Office, Department of Education and Employment, National Assembly for Wales.

Tew, J. (2006) Understanding power and powerlessness: towards a framework for emancipatory practice in social work, *Journal of Social Work*, 6(1): 22–51.

Thomas, K. and Killman, R. (2002) *Thomas-Killman Conflict Mode Instrument*. Mountain View, CA: CPP.

Thompson, N. (2011) *Effective Communication: A Guide for the People Professions*. Basingstoke: Palgrave Macmillan.

Thorpe, A. (2011) The use of power in social work practice, in T. Okitikpi (ed.) *Social Control and the Use of Power in Social Work with Children and Families*. Lyme Regis: Russell House.

Tompsett, H., Ashworth, M., Atkins, C., Bell, L., Gallagher, A., Morgan, M., Neatby, R. and Wainwright, P. (2010) *The Child, the Family and the GP: Tensions and Conflicts of Interest for GPs in Safeguarding Children, May 2006-October 2008*. London: Kingston University.

Travis, A. (2011) UK to deport child asylum seekers to Afghanistan, *The Guardian*, 7 June.

Turnell, A. and Edwards, S. (1997) Aspiring to partnership: the signs of safety approach to child protection, *Child Abuse Review*, 6(3):179–190.

Tyndale, G. (2004) I really believe I am not damaging them by doing this, *The Guardian*, 8 March.

Unicef (2008) *It's about Ability: An Explanation of the Convention on the Rights of Persons with Disabilities*. New York: Unicef.

United Nations (1951) *United Nations Convention Relating to the Status of Refugees*. Available from: http://www.unhcr.org/protect/PROTECTION/3b66c2aa10.pdf [Accessed 22 November 2012].

United Nations (1989) *The United Nations Convention on the Rights of the Child*. Geneva: United Nations.

United Nations Committee on the Rights of the Child (2011) *Fifty Sixth Session Concluding Observations of the Committee on the Rights of the Child: Afghanistan*. Available from: http://www.crin.org/resources/infoDetail.asp?ID=24605&flag=legal [Accessed 22 November 2012].

United Nations Convention on the Rights of Persons with Disabilities (2006) Available from: http://www.un.org/disabilities/documents/convention/convoptprot-e.pdf [Accessed 21 November 2012].

Vojak, C. (2009) Choosing language: social service framing and social justice, *British Journal of Social Work*, 39: 936–949.

Walke, C. (1993) Child protection: the police perspective, in H. Owen and L. Pritchard (eds) *Good Practice in Child Protection: A Manual for Professionals*. London: Jessica Kingsley Publishers.

Walker, J. (2006) *Communication and Social Work from an Attachment Perspective*. Available from: http://jim-walker.co.uk/downloads/Communication%20 and%20social%20work%20from%20an%20attachment%20perspective.pdf [Accessed 9 August 2012].

Watson, N., Shakespeare, T., Cunningham-Burley, S. and Barnes, C. (1999) *Life as a Disabled Child: A Qualitative Study of Young People's Experiences and Perspectives*. Leeds: Disability Research Unit University of Leeds.

Wattam, C. (1996) The social construction of child abuse for practical policy purposes – a review of child protection messages from research, *Child and Family Law Quarterly*, 8(3): 189–200.

Weld, N. (2009) *Making Sure Children get HELD: Ideas and Resources to Help Workers Place Help, Empathy, Love and Dignity at the Heart of Child Protection and Support*. Lyme Regis: Russell House.

White, S. (2008) Drop the deadline. Computers can hinder child protection, *The Guardian*, 19 November.

White, S. (2009) Arguing the case in safeguarding, in K. Broadhurst, C. Grover and J. Jamieson (eds) *Critical Perspectives on Safeguarding Children*. Chichester: Wiley.

Williamson, L. (1998) Unaccompanied but not unsupported, in J. Rutter and C., Jones (eds) *Refugee Education. Mapping the Field*. Stoke on Trent: Trentham Books.

Winter, K. (2011) *Building Relationships and Communicating with Young Children: A Practical Guide for Social Workers*. Oxford: Routledge.

Woodcock Ross, J. (2011) *Specialist Communication Skills for Social Workers*. Basingstoke: Palgrave MacMillan.

WSCB (Wolverhampton Safeguarding Children Board, 2011) *Serious Case Review: Executive Summary Child J*. Wolverhampton: WSCB.

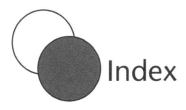

Index

abuse
use of word 28
abuse of power 26
abusive images of children 29–32
accommodation
UASCs 139–40
accountability 62, 65, 68
Achieving Best Evidence (ABE)
guidance 157
Achieving Best Evidence (ABE)
interview
closure 170
free narrative phase 168–9
introduction and rapport phase
167–8
phased interview approach 166
questioning phase 169–70
*Achieving Best Evidence in Criminal
Proceedings: Guidance on
Vulnerable or Intimidated
Witnesses including Children*
165–6
Achieving Best Evidence interview 68,
74
adolescent development 33–7
adult learning disability team 54, 57
adult/child relationship
breaching boundaries of acceptable
25
advocacy 134
Afghanistan
asylum applications from 137–8
UASCs from 137–42
age 97

age disputes
UASCs 141–2
agencies 41, 76, 112, 145, 180
alcohol misuse 100
alienation 118
Alinsky, Saul David [1909–72] 3–4
All Babies Count NSPCC campaign
98
alternative/complementary therapies
149–50
ambiguity 97
ambivalence 102, 134
analysis
balance of intuition and 22–3
Ann Craft Trust Centre for Social
Work 76
appointments
missed 155
approach behaviours 64
approach-avoid axis 64
armed conflict
protection from 137
Aspect
representation and advice from
160
assertiveness 86, 129
assessment 24, 38–9
disabled children 174
Assessment Framework 99
Association of Child Abuse Lawyers
(ACAL) 112
assumptions 118
asylum
definition 138

asylum applications 138–9
Asylum and Immigration Tribunal
   138
asylum seeking children
   unaccompanied 113–46
augmentative communication
   systems 175
augmentative flexibility 63
Australia
   child migrants 184
authenticity 25–7
avoidance 129

background knowledge 22
bearing witness 134
behaviour
   perceived as challenging 101
Bellwood, Simon 147, 184
best interests
   children 154
   maintaining centrality of child's
      150
body language 19
Borders, Citizenship and Immigration
   Act (2009) 139
British Association of Social Workers
   (BASW)
   Code of Ethics 4–5
   representation and advice from 160
bullying 45–7
   disabled children 177

Canada
   child migrants 184
capacity 97
   parental 50
cardiac problems
   obesity related 47, 55
carers
   disabled children 177
case reviews 179
cases
   difficulties in progressing 158–9

change 102
   communication as means of
      achieving 2–4
   inability to force 104
child
   centrality of voice 64–6
   communication with 98
   identity 162
   listening to 101–2
   rights of 98
child abuse 29
   as abuse of power 26
   definition 3
   legal context 32–3
   vulnerability of disabled children
      177
Child Abuse Investigation Team
   (CAIT) 48, 54
child and adolescent mental health
   service (CAMHS) 115, 119,
      121–2
child development 100
Child Exploitation and Online
   Protection Centre (CEOP) 33,
      41
child migrants 184
child murder
   statistics for 100
child in need 148
child pornography
   unacceptability of term 28–9
child protection 39
   barriers to 175
   concerns over procedures for 147
   disabled children 176–8
   enabling engagement 57–8
   proactive 33–7
   raising threshold 148
   shared professional ownership 71
   statutory duty to notify services 67
   threshold for procedures to be
      implemented 67
   whether obesity issue of 67

child protection meetings
  attendance of GPs at 71–2
  key themes 69–70
child protection plans 80
child protection procedures 20
  lack of compliance with 110
child protection register 110
  abolition of 106
child protection teacher 155
child sex offender 30
  use of term 28
child sexual abuse accommodation
    syndrome 31
child sexual exploitation
  investigating 37–40
childhood obesity 44–68
  when becomes child protection
    concern 67
  whether child protection issue
    67
Childhood Obesity National Support
    Team (CONST) 76
childism 184
  disabled children 170–1
children
  asylum seeking 113–46
  ensuring comfort with interviewers
    167
  formal interviews 75
  immigration status 139
  responsibilities of social workers
    183–4
  right to family life 154
  spotlight on crimes against 183
Children Abused Through Sexual
    Exploitation (CATSE) model
    36–7
Children Act (1989) 27, 36–7, 47, 64,
    66, 69, 99, 104, 138–40, 149,
    154, 162
  Section 17 in respect of disabled
    children 174
Children Act (2004) 64, 69–71, 138

Children are Unbeatable Alliance
    112
Children and Families Across Borders
    (CFAB) 145
children first principle 162
children's rights 27
Children's Rights Alliance for England
    (CRAE) 112
Children's Rights Officers and
    Advocates (CROA) 145
children's services
  changing 69–70
Children's Society 141
Chronically Sick and Disabled Persons
    Act (1970) 174
chronology
  creating 104
  example of 105
clarification
  seeking 168
Climbié, Victoria 44, 53, 104
  outcomes from public inquiry into
    murder of 70
  strategy meetings in case of 72–5
closure
  Achieving Best Evidence (ABE)
    interview 170
co-operation 60, 128–9
  illusion of 81
Code of Ethics
  BASW 4–5
codes of practice
  communication within framework
    of 4
cognitive functioning 50
collaboration 60, 129
College of Social Work 1
  Professional Capability Framework 4
collusion 113
communication
  achieving change by 2–4
  barriers to 79, 117
  central to social work 1

with child 98
child's preferred method 175
difficulties in establishing 117
disabled children 171
distorted 23
dynamics of 17
engagement in initial stages 8–9
ethics and values 97–9, 135–7,
    170–2
focusing 78
Johari Window 93–5
judgements about child's 175
knowledge base 28–37, 66–72,
    99–108, 137–42, 172–8
methods 62–4, 95–7, 131–4, 163–70
multi-agency 70
online 9
perpetual screens 92–3
purpose of 60
sufficient time for 176
theory 22–5, 58–60, 62–3, 92–5,
    129–31, 161–3
transmission theory 92
unthreatening and
    non-confrontational context
    for 124–5
values and ethics 64–6
communicative sensitivity 48
complex types of maltreatment
    deciding what constitutes 68–9
compliance 102
complicity 35
compromise 129
concentration
    poor 55
conceptual understanding 25
conceptualization
    within framework of legislation and
        procedure 62
confidence
    in ability to communicate 6
    loss of 19
confidentiality 65

conflict 18–9
    responses to 128–9
conflict resolution 160
confrontation 18
congruence
    lack of 96
Connolly, Peter 79, 97–8
    investigation into death of
        108–11
    death of 71
    outcomes from public inquiry into
        death of 70
consensus decision-making 70
conspiracy
    feelings of 32
constraint 113
Contact a Family 180
containing 134
control 35, 113, 116
conversation 19
Council for Disabled Children 180
crime in progress 29
Criminal Justice and Public Order Act
    (1994) 32
criminal proceedings
    disabled children as witnesses in
        165–6
critical reflection 2
critical witness
    role of 2
cultural advice 136
cultural capital 26, 131

decision-making
    child's role in 64–5
    respectful 62–3
    statutory 67
defensive response 96
defensiveness 104
denial
    children met with 31
dependency 35
    disabled children 177

depression 80–2, 141
deprofessionalization 3
deregulation 147
    social work 1
detention
    UASCs at ports of entry 141
diet 55, 57–8
    management 49
digital cameras
    distribution of indecent images by
        30
disability
    knowledge about specific 172–4
    negative attitudes towards 163
    personal perceptions 164
    social model of 161–2
    terminology of 162
Disability Discrimination Act (2005)
        163
disability teams
    may lack child protection expertise
        162
    role of 162–3
disabled children
    child protection 176–8
    childism 170–1
    communication 171
    discriminatory attitudes towards
        171
    equality of provision 171–2
    ethnic groups 171
    exclusion from child protection
        conferences 172
    family context 176
    family work with 147–81
    intermediaries 178
    isolation experienced by parents
        176
    legislative and policy framework
        174–5
    protection of 149–61
    psychological effects of 153–4
    reluctance to engage with 176

safeguarding 162–3
    services for 162–3
    statistics on 176
    touch 163–4
    vulnerability to child abuse
        176–7
    witnesses in criminal proceedings
        165–6
discretionary leave to remain 137
discrimination
    disabled children 171
distraction 81, 89
dogs
    challenging presence of 82
domestic violence 81
Don't stick it, stop it! campaign 180
drug misuse 100
duty of care 4–5

easy bruising syndrome 80, 84
education social worker
    role of 75
emotional development 49
emotional engagement 134
emotional fragility
    recognising 67
emotional functioning 50
emotional holding 132
emotional impact 119–20
emotional intelligence 58–9, 61–2
emotional issues 136
emotional literacy 60
emotional safety 125
emotional welfare 48
emotions 60
empathy 82, 98, 121
End Child Prostitution, Child
        Pornography and the
        Trafficking of Children for
        Sexual Purposes (ECPAT) 41
engagement 26–7, 36
    initial stages of communication
        8–9

entrapment 10
Equality Act (2010) 174
equality of provision
  disabled children 171–2
ethics 27–8
  communication 64–6, 97–9, 135–7,
    170–2
ethnic groups
  disabled children 171
ethnicity 115
ethnocentrism 129–30
European Convention on Human
    Rights (1950) 138
Every Child in Need 181
exchange model 62–3
exercise 55, 57–8
  lack of 46–7
  management 49
eye contact 132

facial expression 132
false compliance 86, 101–4
false negatives 93
false positives 93
family background
  ascertaining 84–5
Family Centres 80, 89–90
  importance of 86
family home
  discomfort in 89
family support
  intervention by 109
family support model 109
family work
  with disabled children 147–82
fidgeting 132
Foresight Report 66
Forgotten Families 176
foster care 115–6
  shortage of 140
free narrative phase
  Achieving Best Evidence (ABE)
    interview 168–9

friendship networks 14
Friere, Paulo [1921–97] 2–3
frozen watchfulness 97

general practitioners 63
  attendance at child protection
    meetings 71–2
  involvement of 45–9, 51, 55–7,
    157
generation gap 33–4
grooming 10–2, 35
group reasoning 70
guidance
  communication within framework
    of 4

Habermas, Jürgen 23
habitus 130–1
hair
  pulling out own 52, 56
Haringey Local Safeguarding
    Children's Board 109
Haringey, London Borough of
  flaws in child protection 184
  involvement in Victoria Climbié
    case 73–4
Haringey Serious Case Review
  Peter Connolly 98–9
Health and Care Professions Council
    (HCPC) 161
  Standards of Conduct 4–5
  Standards of Proficiency 4–5
health checks
  importance of 84
health concerns 48–9
health information
  public perception of 66–7
Health and Social Care Professionals
    Council 181
health visitors 84
hierarchy
  exaggeration of 50, 107
Hillingdon judgement 139

homeopathy 152
hostility 101
human rights
    achieving for service users 147
    violations 113
Human Rights Act (1998) 138
Humphreys, Margaret 184
hygiene 80–1
hypotheses 22

Ideal Speech Situation 23
identity
    child 162
    confusion over 38
immediacy 95
Immigration Law Practitioner's
    Association (ILPA) 145
immigration policy
    social work and 113
immigration status
    children 139
incident chart
    example of 106
independent facilitators 176
Independent Reviewing Officer (IRO)
    120
information
    collating 104
information sharing
    proportionate 65–6
instability 22
institutional racism 171
integrity 4
intelligence gathering 24
inter agency communication 59
intercultural communication 130
intermediaries
    use with disabled children 178
International Federation of Social
    Work 4
internet access 30
Internet Watch Foundation (IWF) 31,
    41

interpersonal communication
    relationship with intrapersonal
        communication 60
Interpol 33, 41
interpreters 136–7, 176
    use of 75
interruption 85
intervention 19–20, 24, 33–7
interviewers
    ensuring child is comfortable with
        167
interviews
    children on entry to UK 140–1
    controlling 85–6
intimidation 26
    disabled children 177
intrapersonal communication
    relationship with interpersonal
        communication 60
introduction and rapport phase
    Achieving Best Evidence (ABE)
        interview 167–8
intuition
    balance of analysis and 22–3
investigation 24, 78–112
invisible man syndrome 107
iridocyclitis 173
Islington, London Borough of 147
isolation
    disabled children 177
It Matters to Me 41

Jersey
    abuse of young people on 147,
        184
Johari Window 93–5
joint investigations 37–40
judgements 22, 39, 93, 98, 100,
    175
justice
    achieving for users 147
juvenile rheumatoid arthritis
    173

Kemal, Nevres 147, 184
knowledge 2–3
  about disabilities 172–4
  background 22
knowledge base
  communication 28–37, 66–72,
    99–108, 137–42, 172–8

labelling
  disabled children 163
language 115, 136
learning ability 97
learning difficulties 55
  parental 44, 49–50, 52, 56–7, 67
legislation
  communication within framework
    of 4
local authority
  support from 139
local protocols 63
Local Safeguarding Children Board
    71–2, 157, 159–60
London Child Protection Procedures
    28
  relating to disabled children
    177–8
London Safeguarding Children Board
    (LSCB) 112
looked after children 39
loss 127
low self-esteem 34
  obesity related 47

management
  challenging 151–60
medical examinations
  unexplained injuries 90–1
medical findings 73–4
Medical Foundation for the Care of
    Victims of Torture 133–4, 146
medical information
  sharing 53
medical jargon 173–4

medical treatment
  cultural perspectives on 151–2
  resistance to 153–4
medication
  concern over side effects 154
  failure to administer 151, 156
meetings
  key themes of child protection
    69–70
mental health
  asylum seeking children 137
  parental 100
missed opportunities 83
misuse of authority 113
misuse of power
  confronting 2–4
mobile phones
  distribution of indecent images by
    30
mobility
  problems with 149
  stage of 101
monitoring
  accepting 103
MP4 players
  distribution of indecent images by
    30
Multi Agency Planning meetings
    (MAPs) 37
multi-agency networks 36, 93, 148–9
multi-agency process 62, 69–71, 161,
    184
  communication 70
  risk assessment 43–77
multi-agency protection plans 27
multiple disabilities
  increasing risk of abuse 176
Munro Review of Child Protection 158

narrative
  use of 125
National Association of People Abused
    in Childhood (NAPAC) 112

National Coalition of Anti-
  Deportation Campaigns
  (NCADC) 146
National Police Intelligence Agency
  (NPIA) 41
National Society for the Prevention of
  Cruelty to Children (NSPCC)
  30, 112
neglect 79–80, 100
  protection from 78–112
negotiation 43–77
  limiting capacity for 48
  ownership 68
  purpose of 60
network meeting 36–7
networking 3
nightmares 127
noise 49
non-compliance 104
non-leading questions 169
non-verbal behaviour 95, 97
non-verbal communication
  responding to 132–4
nurses 75
nurturance 61

obesity
  childhood 44–68
    when becomes child protection
      concern 67
    whether child protection issue
      67
Office of the Children's Commissioner
  163
Ofsted 110, 161
Ofsted whistleblower hotline 181
omniscient adult effect 133
online abuse of children 30
online communication 9
open questions 96–7
open-ended prompts 168
openness 62
Operation Ore 30

Operation Retriever 38
Operation Span 28
operational targets 24
opportunities
  missed 83
oppression
  disabled children 170–1
optimism
  putting into perspective 100
  the rule of 99–100
oral tradition 133
organizational barriers
  overcoming 147–82
organizational dangerousness 104,
  106–8, 147–8
organized crime 24
ownership 68

paediatric rheumatologists 173
paediatricians 173
  role of 75
paedophile
  use of word 28
pain 149–50
  inability to describe 173
pain relief 173
  withholding 155
paralanguage 117
parental engagement
  withdrawal of 46–7, 67
parental neglect 67
parental resistance 78–112
parenting capacity 179
  assessment for 163
parents
  isolation experienced by of disabled
    children 176
past
  connection with 126
peer relations 54
perpetual screens 92–3
persistence 147–82, 179
  sensitive 121

phased interview approach
   Achieving Best Evidence (ABE)
      interview 166
phatic communication 131–2
photographs
   downloading 16–7
physical ability 97
physical disability
   role of school nurse 149–52
physical harm 79–80, 100–1, 103
   disabled children 177
   protection from 78–112
   triggers 101
planning
   involving child in 125–6
playground violence 45–6
police
   involvement of 20, 48–9, 51–2,
      55–8, 104, 106
   joint investigations 37–40
poor concentration 55
ports of entry
   detention of UASCs at 141
position of trust 30
post disclosure 31
post traumatic stress syndrome 31,
   141
power 26, 65, 113–46
prescribed regulators 161
presumed incompetence 50
priorities
   mixed messages about 118
prioritization 58
privacy 65
privatization 147
procedural guidance 63
Professional Capability Framework
   College of Social Work 4, 97
professional dangerousness 99–101,
   152, 178
professional integrity 183–4
professional language
   changes in 78

professional touch 164
professionals
   avoidance of contact with
      107
protected disclosure 161
Protection of Children Act (1978)
   32
protocols 24
pseudo-photographs 32
psychological hypothermia 133
psychological profiling 32
Public Concern at Work 181
Public Interest Disclosure Act (1998)
   161
Pushtun
   UK community of 137

questioning phase
   Achieving Best Evidence (ABE)
      interview 169–70

R (Behre) v Hillingdon 139
reasoning 60
reflective function 59–61
reflective listening 96
Refugee Children's Consortium (RCC)
   142, 146
Refugee Children's Rights Project
   146
Refugee Council 146
Refugee and Migrant Justice (RMJ)
   135–6, 140–1
relationship-based social work 60
relationships
   building 26
residential care
   crimes against children in 184
Respond 76
responsibilities 75
review strategy meetings 75
right to family life
   children 154
rights of the child 98

risk 36, 150
risk analysis 92–3
risk assessment 21, 67
   multi-agency process 43–77
robustness 68
Rochdale
   sex crimes in 28
rule of optimism 99

*Safe at Last? Children on the Front Line
   of UK Border Control* 144
safe surfing 21
safe working environment 107
safeguarding
   concept of 78
*Safeguarding Disabled Children. Practice
   Guidance* 175
Save the Children 30
Schneider, Betsy 32
school nurse 46–50, 52–3, 56
   role in physical disability 149–52
schoolwork
   deterioration in 47, 55
secrecy 31
Section 47 investigations 20, 27, 47,
   54, 72, 74, 89, 104, 106
   in respect of Peter Connolly murder
   108
Section 47 protocols 99
security 125
Seeing double 97–9
self harm 115–22, 141
self-consciousness 34
self-esteem 38
self-image 36
self-reflection 95
sensitive persistence 121
separation 127
service cuts 69, 147
sexual behaviour
   abusive 28
sexual experimentation
   acceptable 28

sexual exploitation 10, 19
   experiences of 34–5
   indicators of 39
   protection from 9
Sexual Offences Act (2003) 33
sexual risk taking 36
shame 31
sibling relationships 154–5
silence
   responding to 132–4
   use of 120
social activism 1
social development 49
social oppression 184
social services
   initial contact 58
   intervention by 45
social work
   communication central to 1
   disarray of profession 1
   immigration policy and 113
   role of 2
   therapeutic style of 123
   use of power in 113–46
Social Work Action Network (SWAN)
   1
Social Work Reform Board 6
social workers 63
   offering caring relationship within
      clear boundaries 25
   responsibilities towards children
      183–4
   safe working environment for 107
Standards of Conduct, HCPC 4–5
*Standards for Employers of Social
   Workers in England and
   Supervision Framework* 6
Standards of Proficiency, HCPC 4–5
statistics
   child murder 100
statutory duty
   notification regarding child
      protection 67

statutory guidance
   attempts to deregulate 1
stimulation
   lack of 55
Stop It Now 41
storytelling 133–4
strategy meetings 37, 68–9
   pushing for 156–60
Street and Lanes Project 35
street language 133
supervision
   lack of 55
   need for 89
support
   accepting 103
Sure Start programme 44, 54

Talking Mats 164–5
Taylor, Alison 184
terminology
   analysis of 28–9
Three Houses Model 121
time constraints 117
touch
   disabled children 163–4
trade unions
   representation and advice from 160
training
   need for 89
transfer conference 75
transmission theory 92
transparency 68
trust 25–7, 62
type two diabetes
   obesity related 47, 55

UK Border Agency (UKBA) 114,
      138–9
unaccompanied asylum seeking
      children (UASC) 113–46
   age disputes 141–2
   detention at ports of entry 141
   experiences of 142–4

legal and policy context 138–42
   perceptions of 125
unassertiveness 128–9
uncertainty 22
understanding 60
unexplained injuries
   medical examinations 90–1
uniqueness 22
Unison
   representation and advice from
      160
United Kingdom
   entry into 140–1
United Nations Committee on the
      Rights of the Child 137–8
United Nations Convention on the
      Rights of Persons with
      Disabilities (2006) 174
United Nations Convention Relating
      to the Status of Refugees (1951)
      138
United Nations Convention on the
      Rights of the Child (1989) 27,
      32, 64, 174
unsupervised accommodation 139
US Postal Service 30

value conflict 22
values 27–8
   communication 64–6, 97–9, 135–7,
      170–2
victimization 179
Victoria Climbié Inquiry Report
      (2003) 159
Visible Evidence – Forgotten Children 30
visits
   places for 123–5
   to young people 116
vocabulary
   lack of 25
vulnerability 26, 35–6, 39
vulnerable children
   abusive images of 23

vulnerable witnesses
   disabled children in criminal
      proceedings 165–6

welfare cuts 147
whistleblowing 147
   definition 160
Whose Daughter Next? 35
witnesses
   disabled children as in criminal
      proceedings 165–6

Wonderland network 30
Working Together guidance 37, 79,
   104
Working Together procedures 47, 68–9,
   106
Working Together to Safeguard Children
   161, 175
Wright, Lauren
   murder of 71

youth offending plans 39

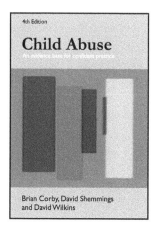

4th Edition

Child Abuse

An evidence base for confident practice

Brian Corby, David Shemmings
and David Wilkins

CHILD ABUSE
An Evidence Base for Confident Practice
Fourth Edition

Brian Corby, David Shemmings and David
Wilkins

9780335245093 (Paperback)
2012

eBook also available

This best-selling text has been used by countless students, practitioners and
researchers as a key reference on child protection issues. The book
demystifies this complex and emotionally-charged area, outlining research,
history, social policy and legislation, as well as the theory and practice
underpinning child protection work.

Key features:

- The latest research and thinking on the causes of child abuse, including
  new insights from the field of attachment theory
- An updated overview of child protection practices, ranging from the 19th
  Century to the • recent 'Baby P' tragedy
- Detailed analysis and coverage of the Munro review of child protection in
  England and the work of the Social Work Reform Board

www.openup.co.uk

OPEN UNIVERSITY PRESS
McGraw - Hill Education